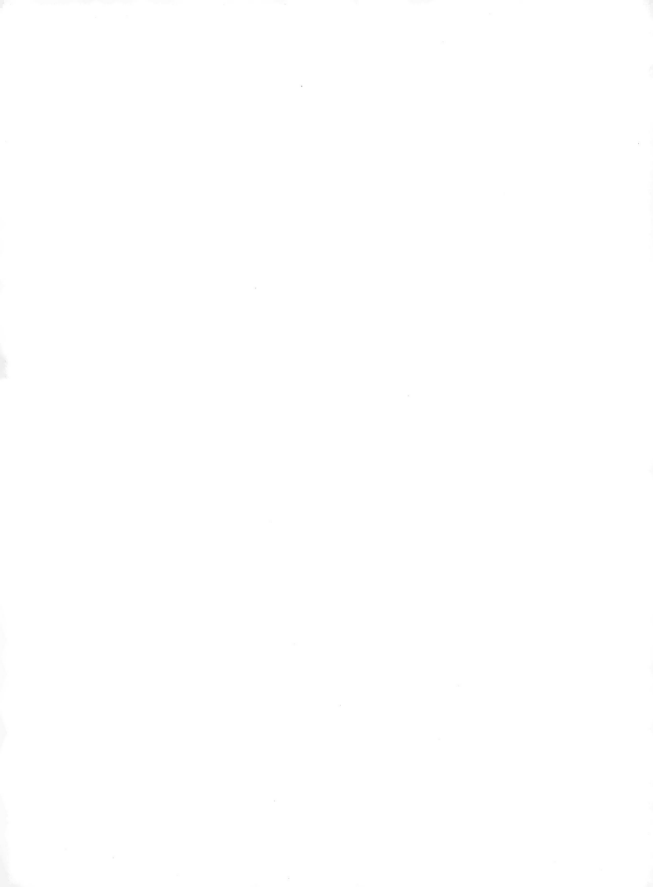

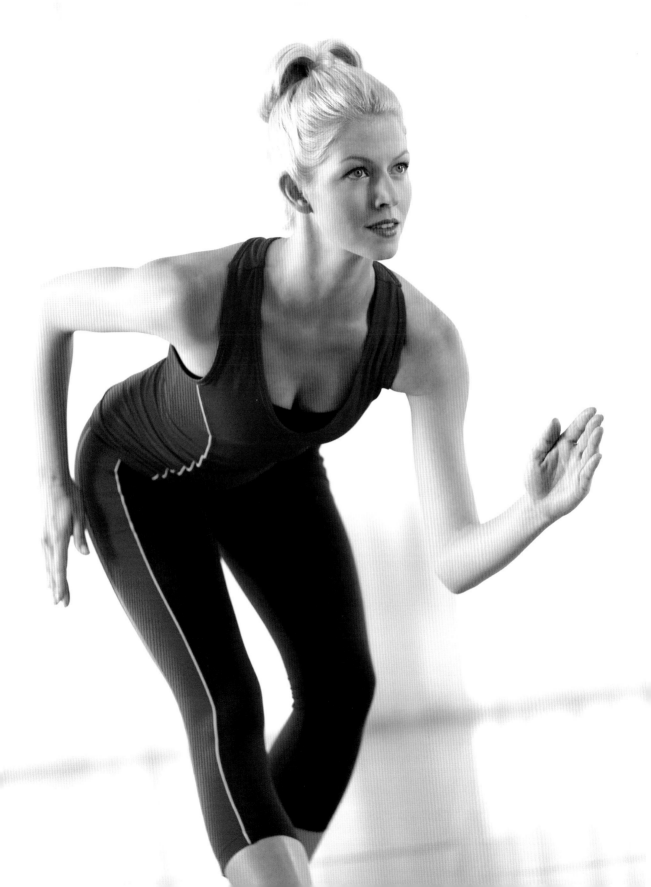

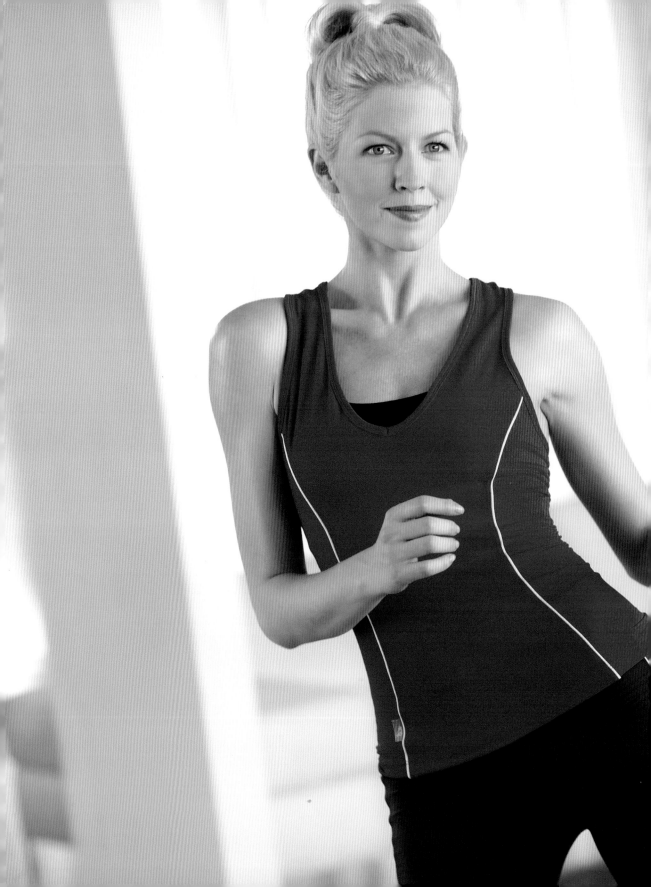

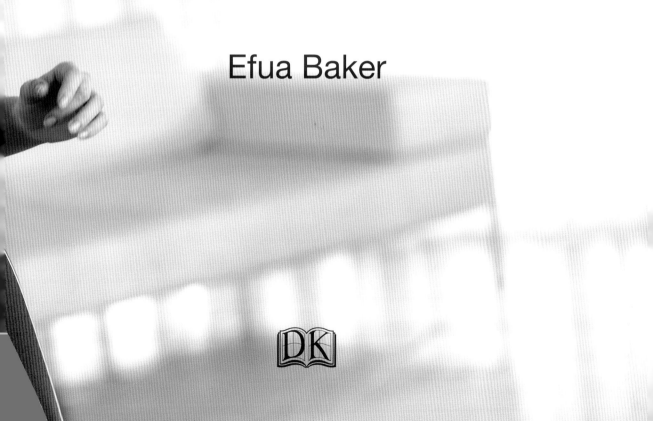

>> **15** minute

calorie burn
workout

Efua Baker

DK

London, New York, Melbourne,
Munich and Delhi

Project Editor Hilary Mandleberg
Project Art Editor Ruth Hope
Senior Editor Jennifer Latham
Senior Art Editor Susan Downing
Managing Editor Dawn Henderson
Managing Art Editor Christine Keilty
Art Director Peter Luff
Publisher Mary-Clare Jerram
Stills Photography Ruth Jenkinson
DTP Designer Sonia Charbonnier
Production Controller Alice Holloway
Senior Production Editor Jennifer Murray

DVD produced for Dorling Kindersley by
Chrome Productions www.chromeproductions.com

Directors Joel Mishcon, Gez Medinger
Producer Hannah Chandler
DOP Benedict Spence, Jon Kassell
Camera Benedict Spence, Jon Kassell
Camera Assistants Mat Hyman, Matt Russell
Gaffer Jonathan Spencer
Production Assistant Sam Rowland
Music Chad Hobson
Voiceover Suzanne Pirret
Voiceover Recording Ben Jones

First published in Great Britain in 2010
by Dorling Kindersley Limited
80 Strand, London WC2R 0RL
Penguin Group (UK)

Health warning
All participants in fitness activities must assume the responsibility for their own actions
and safety. If you have any health problems or medical conditions, consult with your
doctor before undertaking any of the activities set out in this book. The information
contained in this book cannot replace sound judgement and good decision making,
which can help reduce risk of injury.

A CIP catalogue record is available from the British Library

ISBN 978-1-4053-4417–3

Printed and bound by Sheck Wah Tong Printing Press Ltd, China

Discover more at
www.dk.com

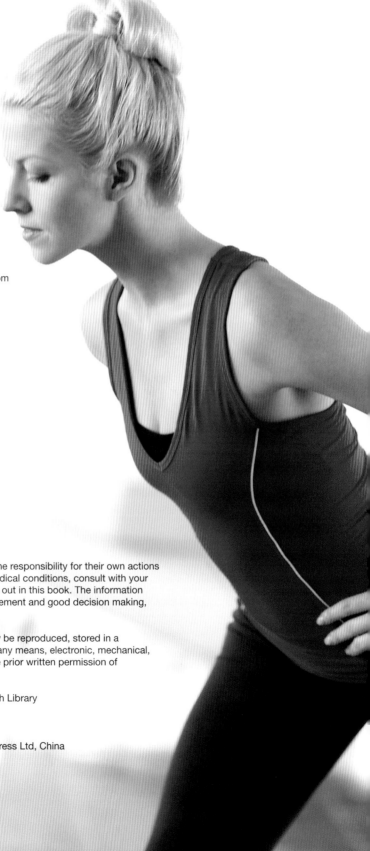

contents

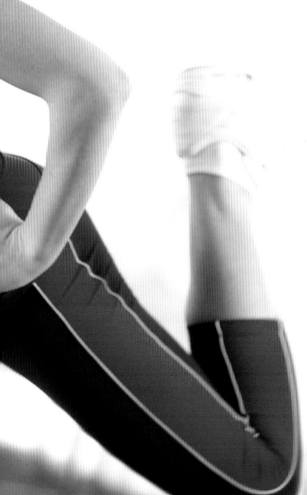

author foreword

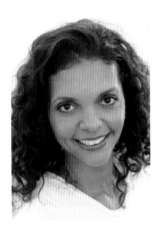

I've always been fascinated with training, or "body sculpting", which is the term I use to describe what I do. It still amazes me how much you can alter the human body by what you feed it and how you train it. I've worked with clients who've lost huge amounts of weight and have radically changed their shape. They've achieved, literally, "miracle" results. And how? By doing the right workouts and eating the right foods. That's it.

If there were some pill we could take that would give us a "six-pack" or keep our body toned and gorgeous without needing to do any workouts, we'd all be strutting around with flawless, perfect bodies. We're not. There isn't such a pill. So ...

You need to take in less fuel (calories) than you use in order to lose weight. If you take in more fuel (calories) than you use, you'll store it as fat and gain weight. Rocket science? New breakthrough discovery? No, just the boring facts.

We all know what we need to do. We just need to do it! Eat sensibly and get moving. The key to keeping it all going is building little changes into your daily routine so it doesn't feel like a diet, or a programme, or a drag. Most importantly, you need to find a type of movement that you really enjoy doing, something you get a "buzz" out of. That way you'll keep on doing it. This book offers you four different styles of workout that will burn calories. Try them all and hopefully find at least one that suits you. That way you can actually enjoy getting rid of that excess fuel.

I'm a great believer in being proactive and making changes when things aren't working. What's great with diet and exercise, unlike so many other things in life, is that you can be in complete control and can reap all the benefits yourself. If you're not happy with the size or shape of your butt, get started burning calories and sculpting muscle now. Do something about it. I'm here and happy to help you!

sweaty**Betty** foreword

It is my belief that women can feel empowered through fitness.

Before I opened the first sweatyBetty boutique in London's trendy Notting Hill I had no major commitments. Outside of my 9 to 5 job my time was my own and keeping fit and healthy was fun and easy. Nowadays, with a husband, three kids, and a whole chain of boutiques to look after, I have very little "me" time!

I'm the first to admit that finding the time to work out can be a challenge but it's essential if, like me, you need to juggle your work and home life. So whilst I'm unlikely to run a marathon, swim the Channel, or climb Everest in the near future, I can certainly do enough to keep myself looking and feeling good.

We can all find a spare 15 minutes, a few times a week, in the comfort of our own home to keep our bodies and minds in check. So I encourage you to get off the sofa and get active, in sweatyBetty gear of course…!

Tamara Hill-Norton

Founder of sweatyBetty
the UK's leading women's activewear retailer

>> **how to** use this book

Boxing, aerobics, running, or dancing. You choose. Each and every one of these fabulous 15-minute workouts will help you to burn calories and re-shape, sculpt, and tone your body. They're all inspiring and great fun to do, so just pick one – and start moving!

Each of the four programmes in this book and DVD gives you a self-contained 15-minute workout that will burn calories and help shape and tone your body. The DVD has been designed to accompany the book. As you watch it, page references to the book will flash up on the screen. You can refer to the book for more detailed instruction.

In all the workouts, you will usually repeat the move four times, or a multiple of four times. For example, you may do a movement four times to the right followed by four times to the left, or you may alternate sides eight times.

Of the four programmes, the boxing and running sequences are slightly more strenuous than the other two, but it's easy to bring the level of intensity down a notch by modifying some of the movements (see p16). Just go ahead and start with the programme that most interests you.

The number of calories you'll burn when you do the programmes will depend a lot on your personal body type and general level of fitness and activity. Look out for the tips on how to maximize your efforts (see pp16–17) and get the most into, and out of, your 15 minutes.

The gatefolds

The gatefolds are a series of small pictures that offer a summary of each programme. They will come in handy once you have a good grasp of the workout you are doing. Use them for easy reference or as a reminder of the next move you should do.

Safety issues

Always be sensible when exercising. If you're feeling good, then great. Push yourself a little. If you aren't, reduce the level of intensity you are working at (see Talk Test, p14). Remember, it is always wise to consult your health practitioner before starting any exercise programme, particularly if you are suffering from any injuries or illness, or if you are taking any long-term medication.

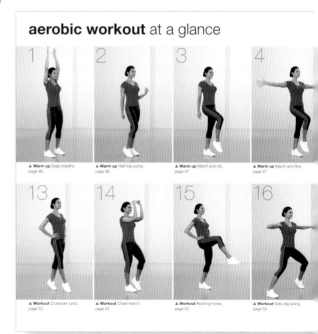

aerobic workout at a glance

▲ **Warm up** Deep breaths, page 46
▲ **Warm up** Half-toe pump, page 46
▲ **Warm up** March and roll, page 47
▲ **Warm up** March and flick, page 47

▲ **Workout** Crossover jump, page 52
▲ **Workout** Chest march, page 52
▲ **Workout** Rocking horse, page 53
▲ **Workout** Side-dig swing, page 53

Gatefold A quick glance at the gatefold summaries at the end of each section provides a reminder of the sequence and of proper form.

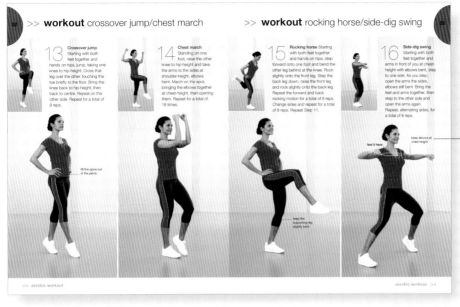

13 **Crossover jump** Starting with both feet together and hands on hips, jump, taking one knee to hip-height. Cross that leg over the other, touching the toe briefly to the floor. Bring the knee back to centre. Repeat on the other side. Repeat for a total of 8 reps.

14 **Chest march** Standing on one foot, raise the other knee to hip-height and take the arms to the sides at shoulder-height, elbows bent. March on the spot, bringing the elbows together at chest-height, then opening them. Repeat for a total of 16 times.

15 **Rocking horse** Starting with both feet together and hands on hips, step forward onto one foot and bend the other leg behind at the knee. Rock slightly onto the front leg. Step the back leg down, raise the front leg and rock slightly onto the back leg. Repeat the forward and back rocking motion for a total of 8 reps. Change sides and repeat for a total of 8 reps. Repeat Step 11.

16 **Side-dig swing** Starting with both feet together and arms in front of you at chest-height with elbows bent, step to one side. As you step, open the arms to the sides, elbows still bent. Bring the feet and arms together, then step to the other side and open the arms again. Repeat, alternating sides, for a total of 8 reps.

lift the spine out of the pelvis

keep the supporting leg slightly bent

feel it here

keep elbows at chest height

annotations provide extra cues, tips, and insights

>> aerobic workout

aerobic workout >>

Step-by-step pages The inset photograph at the upper left gives you the starting position for the exercise, where necessary. The large photograph gives you the step required to complete it.

the gatefold shows all the exercises in the programme

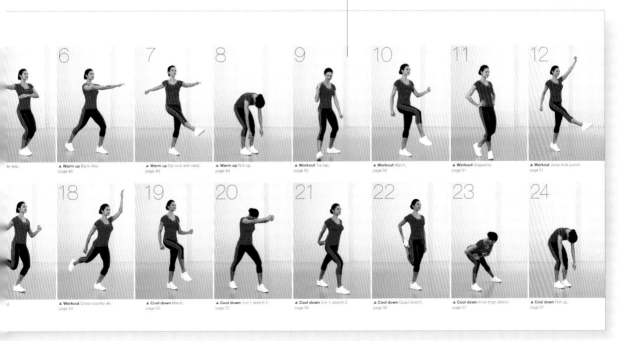

de step.

6 ▲ **Warm up** Back step, page 48

7 ▲ **Warm up** Dip-kick with twist, page 49

8 ▲ **Warm up** Roll-up, page 49

9 ▲ **Workout** Toe tap, page 50

10 ▲ **Workout** March, page 50

11 ▲ **Workout** Grapevine, page 51

12 ▲ **Workout** Jump-kick punch, page 51

18 ▲ **Workout** Cross-country ski, page 54

19 ▲ **Cool down** March, page 55

20 ▲ **Cool down** 3-in-1 stretch 1, page 55

21 ▲ **Cool down** 3-in-1 stretch 2, page 56

22 ▲ **Cool down** Quad stretch, page 56

23 ▲ **Cool down** Inner-thigh stretch, page 57

24 ▲ **Cool down** Roll-up, page 57

>> **what** are calories?

Calories are units of energy. They provide the fuel we need for our body to function – to keep our heart beating, for breathing, for digestion, for making new blood cells, and for maintaining our body temperature. They also provide us with the fuel for moving and exercising.

We get our calories from the food we eat, just as a car gets its power from petrol. Unfortunately, unlike a car, we don't have a limited amount of space – the petrol tank – to store fuel that isn't used immediately. Bodies are very accommodating. They will store any excess fuel (calories) in case of a famine. The problem is that this excess is stored in the form of fat around our bodies.

All we need to do, it seems, is to "balance the books". Take in roughly as much fuel as we use and – voilà – no spare fuel tanks required!

So how much energy *do* we use? To maintain a healthy body weight, women require an average of 2200 calories per day and men 2500 calories. But to find how much you need as an individual is not straightforward. Your Basal Metabolic Rate (BMR)

CALCULATING YOUR DAILY CALORIE REQUIREMENT

To work out your daily calorie requirement, you first need to find your Basal Metabolic Rate (BMR) – the amount of energy your body needs to maintain itself. This accounts for 50 to 80 per cent of your total energy use. The rest of the energy you need is for your muscles to work as you move in your daily life. That varies according to your level of activity and whether you are a man or a woman.
Note: 1in = 2.54cm; 1kg = 2.2lb

Men's BMR = 66 + (13.7 x weight in kg) + (5 x height in cm) – (6.8 x age in years)

Women's BMR = 655 + (9.6 x weight in kg) + (1.8 x height in cm) – (4.7 x age in years)
So if you're female, 30 years old, 167.6cm tall (5ft 6in), and weigh 54.5kg (120lb), your BMR =
655 + 523 + 302 – 141 = 1339 calories/day

Now that you know your BMR, you can work out your **daily calorie requirement** by using the chart below:
So if your BMR is 1339 calories per day, and you are moderately active, your daily calorie requirement =
1.55 x 1339 = 2075 calories/day

ACTIVITY LEVEL	BMR		
If you're sedentary (little or no exercise, desk job)	BMR	x	1.2
Gently active (light exercise/sports 1–3 days a week)	BMR	x	1.375
Moderately active (moderate exercise/sports 3–5 days a week)	BMR	x	1.55
Very active (hard exercise/sports 6–7 days a week)	BMR	x	1.725
Extra active (hard daily exercise/sports and physical job)	BMR	x	1.9

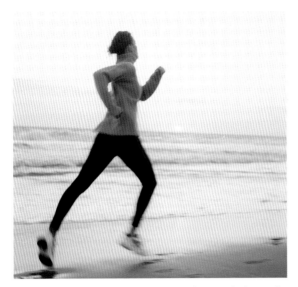

Going out for a run is a great way to burn calories and a chance to get out in the fresh air. You can run off a juicy 150 calories with just 15 minutes' running.

is the amount of energy your body needs to function at rest, but we all burn/use calories at different rates. Your BMR is influenced by your age, sex, lean-muscle-to-fat ratio (a lean, muscular person will burn more calories than someone with a higher proportion of fat, even while sleeping), and your genetic package. The table opposite shows you how to calculate your daily calorie requirement. If you eat more than this, and don't move more, then you are simply going to get fat!

Let's say you want to lose 3.5kg (7lb). To get rid of just 0.5kg (1lb) of excess fat you must burn off around 3500 calories. Of course, you can pare down what you eat (and eating little and often also helps burn calories) but if you go for a two-pronged attack – diet *and* exercise – you have a much better chance of success. It's simple. Take in less fuel, burn more off. What is more, exercise will help build muscle which, in turn, will burn more fat.

So, what sort of exercise helps to burn the calories? Any exercise is better than none, but it's generally accepted that the best is aerobic exercise. This means working your cardiovascular system – the heart and lungs – by doing continuous, rhythmic exercise using large muscle

HOW MANY CALORIES CAN I BURN?

Whether you're exercising or simply doing household chores, you're always burning calories. This chart shows you how many, on average, a person weighing 70kg (155lb) burns doing each activity for 15 minutes. The calories burned vary according to your age, weight, level of fitness, and how hard you exercise.

DO THIS FOR 15 MINUTES	KCALS BURNED
Skipping with a rope	185
Boxing with a partner	165
Running (8kph/5mph)	150
Cross-country skiing	149
Cycling (20kph/12.5mph)	149
High-impact aerobics	130
Downhill skiing	111
Swimming	110
Shovelling snow	110
Low-impact aerobics	100
Dancing	100
Gardening	83
Childcare	65
Raking the lawn	60
Cooking	46
Sitting in a meeting	30
Working at the computer	26
Watching TV	14
Sleeping	11

groups. All the sequences in this book are aerobic, so following them is the best place to start, but the chart above shows how many calories you can burn doing different forms of exercise.

As well as knowing how many calories I burn when I exercise, I also like to have an idea of the calorific value of the foods I eat. Eating a chocolate shortcake cookie means I need to do 15 minutes of low-impact aerobics to compensate. Hmmm ...

>> the **motivation** game

Different things motivate different people to get fit, so first and foremost, it's essential to find the key to start your engine! If you're not clear why exercise is important, read on and discover that, whatever your reasons for exercising, the benefits can't be beaten.

For most of the people I work with, looking good is their main reason for hiring me as their body sculptor. This may be what motivates you, too, whether you're aiming for a bikini holiday, a wedding, or simply to have your friends remark on how great you're looking lately.

It's true that there are more important, health-related reasons for exercising (see opposite), but there's no denying that for a lot of people, physical appearance is their number one motivation. And that's okay. Because the positive side effects of exercising on a regular basis are manifold – you'll be looking and feeling better, because your body is becoming fitter and healthier.

Finding exercise you enjoy means you are more likely to stay motivated. Exercising with a friend helps, too. You wouldn't want to let your friend down, would you?

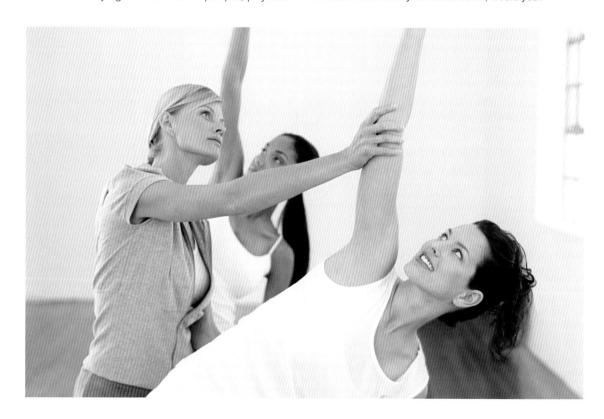

Then there's another category of people who turn to exercise because they're finding that things they could do without thinking 10 or 20 years ago are much harder. Suddenly, gardening, housework, or doing a favourite sport aren't as easy as they once were. For these people, exercise is a route to becoming strong and supple enough to carry on doing the things they've always done.

The health benefits

We all know more or less what we could be doing to benefit our bodies. Regular exercise promotes better cardiovascular and respiratory function. Studies have shown, beyond doubt, that it reduces the risks of coronary heart disease, lowers blood pressure, and also increases levels of "good" cholesterol. It helps control blood-sugar levels and so prevents or controls diabetes. It also improves bone density, which protects against osteoporosis. What is more, exercise can help delay some of the physiological effects of ageing and creates beneficial changes in the metabolism of the body, for instance speeding up the rate at which it burns calories (see p10).

Additionally, exercise helps to combat sleep disorders such as insomnia, and it brings psychological benefits, too, for instance releasing stress and improving self-confidence. These days exercise is frequently prescribed for patients with depression, and can be as effective as some anti-depressant medications. On top of that, regular exercise is linked to better sexual function and an increased sex drive.

Working out regularly promotes stronger bones, flexible muscles, better posture and breathing function, and a generally more efficient body – all of which means you will look better. And we all know that it's easier to relate to results we can see, such as improved muscle tone or weight loss, than to "invisible" improvements in cholesterol, blood pressure, and bone-density levels. However, remember you will be reaping benefits in those areas, too, as a bonus, whether you are interested in them or not. So what on earth are you waiting for? Start exercising!

>> top tips to stay motivated

- **Find a form of exercise** you enjoy so you'll be sure to look forward to it. There are so many different types on offer, there's bound to be one for you.

- **Results are key**, so take advice (and read this book) to find out what exercise gives fast, lasting results. Once you see your body change for the better, it will reduce your chances of giving up.

- **Training for a particular event** is a great way to stay on track. Fun runs and mini triathlons are ideal for helping you to stay focused as you work towards the big day.

- **Keep your body on its toes.** Like you, your body loves variety, so make small changes in your workout from time to time. That keeps *you* interested and wakes your body up and helps it to burn more calories.

- **Stopped seeing results?** Change your programme, try a different class, or work with a different piece of equipment. Just as small changes in your workout can give your body a jump-start, so a complete change is as good as a full engine clean.

- **Use a personal trainer.** Seeing a personal trainer, even if it's just once or twice so they can design a personalized plan for you, can give you a boost and accelerate your progress once you are up and running.

- **Work with a friend.** If you train with an exercise buddy, you'll find it that much harder to skip a session than if you're home alone.

- **If finding even 15 minutes** a day is beyond you right now, work some extra actiivity into your life. Try gardening, walking part of the way to work, or cycling.

>> **let's exercise** safely

Congratulations! You've decided to get your body moving, burn some calories, slim yourself down, and be more healthy. But if you're new to exercise, it's important to know how to work out safely, so follow my tips and you won't suffer any exercise-related injuries.

I've already flagged up what to do if you have any health problems or are taking long-term medication (see p8), but once you're ready to exercise, it's extremely important to stay safe and avoid problems before they happen. Here are some key "Do's" and "Dont's".

Do always warm up. The amount and type of warming up you need depends on what exercise or sport you're going to do, so you'd walk to warm up before you go jogging, and you'd jog before you go running. Your warm up also depends on your personal fitness profile, including your age and any

past injuries. The older you are, the less cushioning there is in your joints to lubricate and protect them, so you'll need longer to prepare your body for exercise. When it comes to previous injuries, you'll want to pay extra attention to warming up the injured area. Climate is something else that affects your warm up. If you are in a cold environment, it will take longer for your muscles to get warm and ready to work than if you are somewhere warm.

Don't skip your cool down stretches. A cool down gradually lowers your heart rate, body temperature, and rate of breathing. It prevents dizziness, stops your blood from suddenly pooling in your hands and feet, and instead gets it circulating properly throughout your body. A cool down can be a slower or lower-intensity version of the exercise you've just done. In the case of my *15 Minute Calorie Burn Workout*, the cool down starts with a March, and moves on to stretches. Apart from helping to prevent injuries, stretching at the end of your workout decreases any tightening you may feel in your muscles after you've finished.

Do make sure you have the right footwear for your activity. This doesn't have to be anything fancy or expensive, but it must be sensible. There are plenty of shoes on the market that look like trainers but are just fashion footwear. These won't support your feet during a workout. For the sequences in this book, you'll need a good pair of cross trainers. Your footwear is especially important if you are doing high-impact exercise like running, so for that you must buy special running shoes.

>> **the talk** test

- **If talking is easy** while you're doing light activity, then you aren't exercising enough.

- **If you can talk comfortably** while you're doing moderate activity, then you're exercising at a good rate.

- **If talking is a little more difficult** and you're doing vigorous activity, then this is still a good rate of exercise for you.

- **If you can't talk** because you're short of breath while doing vigorous activity, then you're working too hard. Slow down.

Don't set unrealistic goals and disappoint yourself. When doing these workouts, you may find that your first goal is simply to get through the warm up in time to the music. Then you can build up from there.

Do invest in a good-fitting sports bra. It doesn't matter if you are not particularly well endowed in the bust department, you can cause irreparable damage to the ligaments that support your bust if you pound away with no support – even if it's just for 15 minutes.

Don't rush into exercise. Start gently and pace yourself. Most exercise-related injuries are caused by people pushing too hard when they're starting out. You're not going to be running a marathon or climbing Mount Everest after just a week's effort.

Do maintain good form and posture at all times during your exercise. If you can't maintain a straight, well-lifted back, pulled-in tummy, and relaxed shoulders (see p16), you aren't working correctly, won't burn so many calories, and have much more chance of sustaining an injury or of creating or aggravating any postural imbalances.

Don't exercise if you're feeling unwell, or after drinking alcohol. You won't be sufficiently in tune with your body, and won't be able to exercise safely and correctly.

Do vary and adapt your workout. Your results will slow down – or "plateau" – if you stick to the exact same workout and level of intensity (see p13).

Stretching after exercise helps prevent injuries. This floor version of the Quad stretch (see p32) is useful if you can't keep your balance when standing. Cushion your hips.

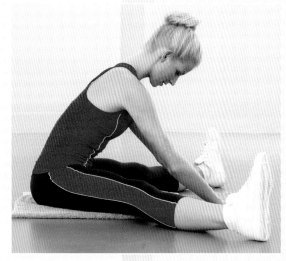

Don't skip your cool down. If you can't manage the Inner-thigh stretch (see p33), try this alternative sitting on the floor. Use padding under your bottom to help you lift your back.

Don't eat unhealthily. Your body can only function well if you give it top-quality fuel. That means a balanced mix of protein, carbohydrates, and fats (see p121).

Do drink plenty. When you are exercising properly, you should sweat, so drink half a glass of water at 10- to 15-minute intervals to replace the fluid you lose through sweating.

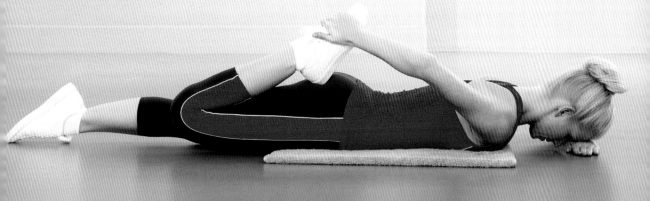

>> **personalize** your exercise

Your *15 Minute Calorie Burn Workout* is hopefully just a start. Read on if you want to burn calories even faster or to learn how to tone things down if you're out of condition or are having an off-day. My tips show the way and – even better – they can be applied to almost any exercise.

If you're going to the trouble of taking 15 minutes out of your day to follow my workouts, then it makes sense to try to maximize your results. It's natural to ask how you can burn even more calories in 15 minutes, especially if you find it hard to resist the occasional sweet treat the rest of the time. Also, as you progress with your exercise, you may discover that you reach a "plateau" (see p13). This is because your body cleverly adjusts to your level of work and decides to take a holiday. You need to give it a wake-up call from time to time.

You'll be glad to know that there are plenty of ways of intensifying your exercise, both to burn more calories in the time available and to get yourself off the "plateau".

Flawless form

Firstly, remind yourself to work with flawless form all the time. That means holding your tummy in, keeping your back straight, and keeping your shoulders relaxed. It's not as easy as it sounds, and it's precisely for that reason that you'll burn more calories. Think of the effort it takes just to keep your tummy in. That effort translates into more calories burned. Not only that, but working your muscles harder means that they become sleek and toned that much faster.

Practising a technique descriptively titled "mind to muscle" will help you work with flawless form. Simply focus on the area you want to feel working, and try to channel your muscle tension and effort on that area. At the same time make a conscious

effort to relax any other part of your body you feel is trying to "join in". This may sound very simple, but if you master this technique you are without a doubt going to get a lot more out of your training.

Max your moves

Next, it pays to put all you've got into each move. When you're marching, lift your knees high and really swing your arms. If you're jogging, pick your

---

>> **taking it** down a notch

- **Go from high-impact to low-impact.** If you're doing the Jog (pp54, 74), bring it down to the level of the March (pp50, 74). If you're doing the Skip (p26), do the March.

- **Omit the hops and jumps.** If you're getting out of breath, simply take a step instead of doing a hop or a jump.

- **Bring your arms down.** Raising your hands above your head increases your heart rate, so if it's getting too much, take them down and concentrate on maintaining good form and the footwork.

- **Do your cool down stretches on the floor.** If you're exhausted at the end of a workout, don't skip your cool down, but stretch on the floor instead (see p15).

feet up and focus on springing off the floor. Intensify any side-to-side steps by making those steps bigger. Exaggerate all the up-down movements. Punch and kick with power. Any and all of these will burn off just a few extra calories and you'll quickly find that they add up.

Add some weight

Another tip is to get yourself a pair of small handweights and do the workouts holding those. If you find that awkward, you can wear weighted fingerless gloves instead. Start with a very light weight, say, 250g–500g (8oz–1lb) in/on each hand. Follow the workout and you'll be surprised how heavy those dinky little weights start to feel. Don't be put off by that. The weights are what make you work harder and burn calories faster. They will also give you fabulously toned arms. When you work with weights, be careful to maintain your form throughout, and if you can't manage that, then just put the weights down for a while.

Extend your workout

Last but not least, if you're prepared to work for more than your allotted 15 minutes, there's no reason – as long as you can still do the Talk Test (see p14) – why you can't lengthen your workout. You could double up on the number of reps you do for each step, you could repeat the entire workout again, from Step 9 to Step 18, or you could follow Step 9 to Step 18 from one workout with Step 9 to Step 18 from another. Just remember to always start with a warm up (Steps 1 to 8), and finish with a cool down (Steps 19 to 24).

Burn off extra calories by doing the routines holding handweights. The extra weight makes your body work harder, and you'll get fabulous arms at the same time.

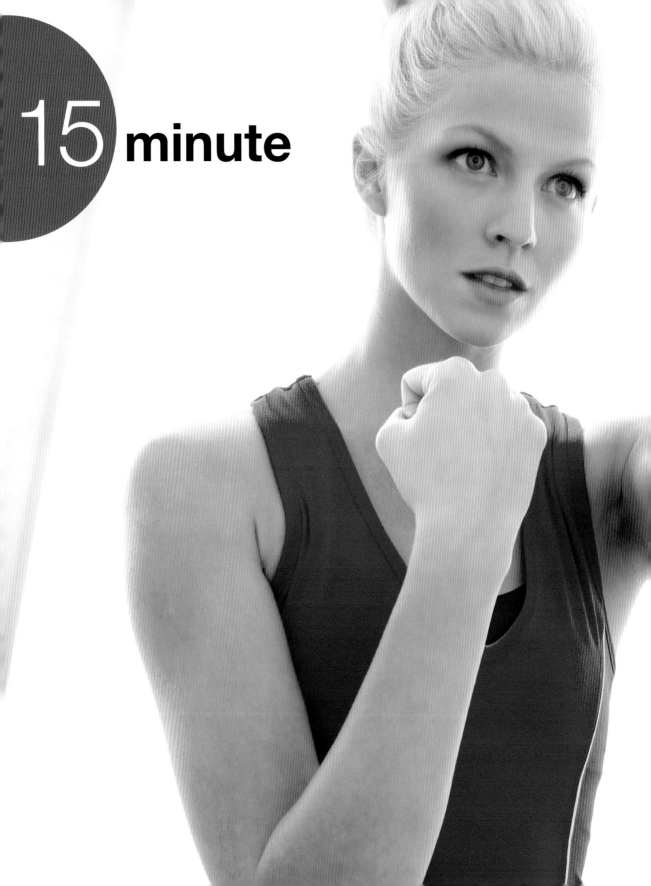

15 minute

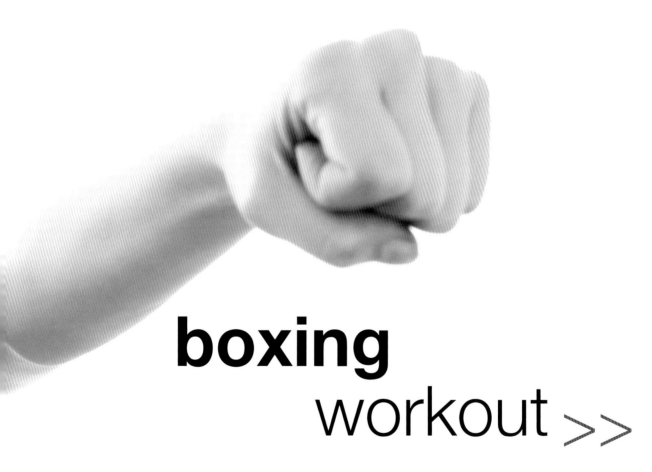

boxing
workout >>

Box your way to a leaner,
more powerful physique.
Strengthen and tone the body.
Focus the mind.

>> **boxing** workout

The various styles of boxing give the most intense all-over body training I have ever tried. This is one of the more demanding workouts in the book, blending the two styles – boxing and kickboxing. It's a great stress reliever, as well as a way of wringing maximum calories out of your 15 minutes.

Boxing and kickboxing are becoming increasingly popular, particularly with women. This type of exercise is fun but challenging. The aerobic element will help you to sculpt your body and burn calories, while the coordination, power, and balance that all types of boxing training offer are undeniably empowering and can be great for your self-confidence, too.

My workout includes kicking, punching, ducking, and skipping. It is not only one of the most effective for stripping off unwanted weight, but you'd be hard pushed to find a muscle group that this sequence doesn't work.

Let's start with your abs. Although my sequence doesn't include any traditional sit-ups, it offers a great abdominal workout. As long as you maintain good form and posture, and really work on keeping your tummy pulled in (without holding your breath), you can achieve more than you think.

The various kicks are also great for working the abs. Once you have engaged the abs – isolated them and got them working – imagine your legs are being lifted by them as if on puppet strings. That makes you work from your centre. It also helps relax the front of your thighs (the quads), which can take over and dominate if you're not careful.

The biceps and chest muscles will also get a good workout. While performing jabs and punches, you need to pay attention to keeping your shoulders down and relaxed. We're not trying to work your neck. Focus on the work of your biceps and chest muscles instead.

> >> **tips for** my boxing workout
>
> - Maintain "mind to muscle" focus (see p16). When punching, focus on the biceps; when kicking, focus on your bottom and legs. Your abs should be "on" throughout.
>
> - Mimic a proper skipping action, making small circular movements with your hands as if you were turning a skipping rope. You'll know you're doing it correctly when you feel it in your biceps.
>
> - This is a demanding workout, but worth mastering. Practice makes perfect, so don't be discouraged when you start.

Remember, too, that it's a lot harder actually punching or kicking something than punching or kicking into space. So, you need to strike into the air as hard as you can to maintain an element of power in your arms and legs.

This workout is designed to burn calories and tone muscles, but you'll also improve your coordination and focus, and it's a fantastic way to let off steam!

Your boxing workout exercises many of your muscle groups, and encourages coordination of the body, while helping you to generate power and balance.

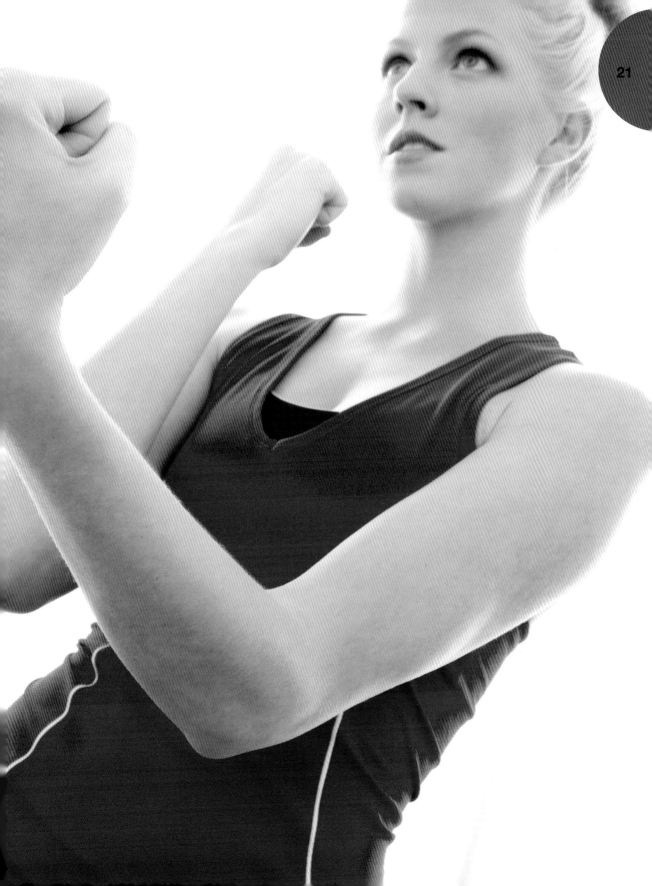

>> **warm up** deep breaths/half-toe pump

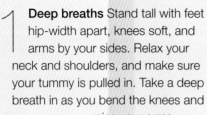

1 **Deep breaths** Stand tall with feet hip-width apart, knees soft, and arms by your sides. Relax your neck and shoulders, and make sure your tummy is pulled in. Take a deep breath in as you bend the knees and raise your arms above your head. Exhale as you lower them with a smooth circular movement. Make sure your back stays straight. Repeat for a total of 4 reps.

to really lengthen your spine, lift from the hips as you raise the arms upwards

2 **Half-toe pump** Alternate your weight from one foot to the other, rising up onto the ball of your foot. As you alternate feet, curl the opposite arm to your shoulder. Keep your hands in a loose fist and make sure you push your heel right down to the floor as you work your calf muscle. Repeat for a total of 16 reps (1 rep = both sides/directions).

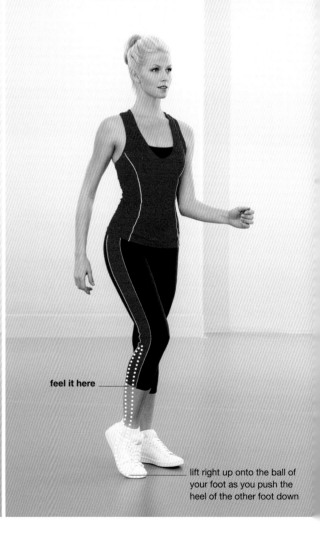

feel it here

lift right up onto the ball of your foot as you push the heel of the other foot down

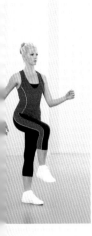

3 **March and roll** Standing on one foot, raise the other knee to waist-height. At the same time, raise the opposite arm. March on the spot, raising opposite knees and arms. Repeat for a total of 8 reps. Then, with your arms by your sides, raise your shoulders towards your ears and roll them in a circular motion, backwards, then forwards. Repeat for a total of 4 reps.

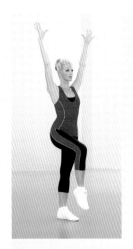

4 **March and flick** Continue marching and, as you do so, stretch your arms sideways to meet above your head, opening and closing your hands at intervals with a "flicking" motion, to warm your fingers and wrists. Continue "flicking" your hands as you lower your arms. Repeat for a total of 4 reps.

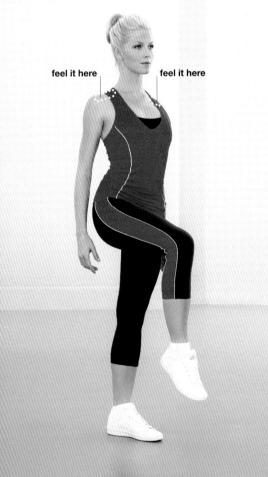

feel it here   feel it here

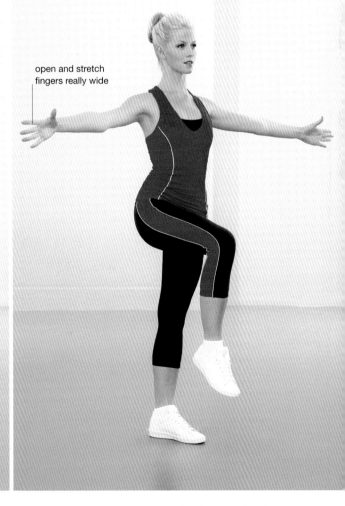

open and stretch fingers really wide

>> **warm up** side step/back step

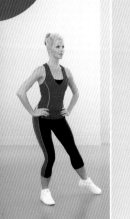

5 **Side step** With hands on hips, take a step to one side, then bring your feet together. Repeat to the other side. Repeat for a total of 4 reps, then swing your arms in the same direction as you are stepping. Your arms should be relaxed and raised no higher than shoulder-height. Repeat for a total of 8 reps.

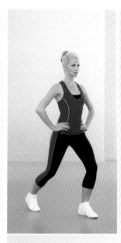

6 **Back step** With hands on hips, touch one foot on the floor behind you. Return to centre and repeat with the opposite foot. Keep your weight centred as you alternate legs. Repeat for a total of 4 reps, then add an arm push in time with your leg movements by pushing both arms forward and back just below shoulder-height. Repeat for a total of 8 reps.

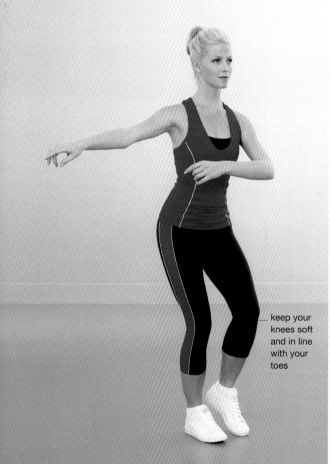

keep your knees soft and in line with your toes

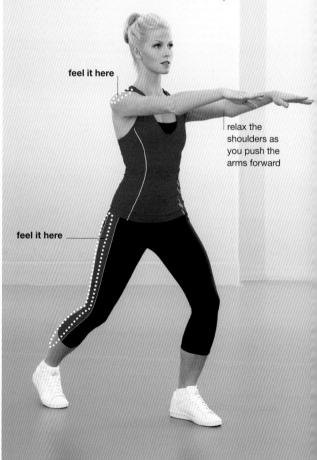

feel it here

relax the shoulders as you push the arms forward

feel it here

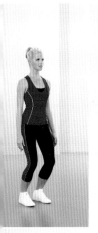

7 **Dip-kick with twist** With arms by your sides, bend both knees, then come up and kick one foot forward. Repeat for a total of 8 reps, then add a twist by turning your upper body and swinging the opposite arm to the kicking leg. Keep the arms shoulder-height. Keep your hips square. Repeat, alternating sides, for a total of 8 reps.

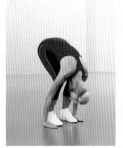

8 **Roll-up** Stand tall with feet hip-width apart, arms stretched above your head, shoulders relaxed, and neck and spine in line. Slowly lower your arms and take your chin towards your chest, then round your back and slowly bend down towards the floor. When you are as low as possible, your hands should be relaxed and as near to the floor as is comfortable. Take a deep breath into your lower back. Then, keeping your tummy pulled into your lower back, uncurl slowly, one vertebra at a time, until you have returned to a standing position.

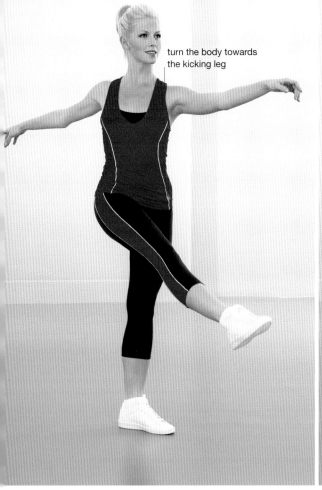

turn the body towards the kicking leg

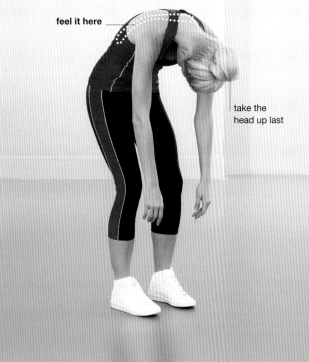

feel it here

take the head up last

>> **workout** punch across/skip

9 **Punch across** Standing with your feet slightly wider than hip-width apart, knees soft and pointing forward, punch one arm across your body for a total of 8 times, keeping the other fist tucked under your chin. Punch with the fist facing down. Repeat on the opposite side then, keeping your lower body in the same position, punch across your body, alternating sides for a total of 8 reps.

10 **Skip** Bring your feet together, arms by your sides, and "skip" with an imaginary rope, alternating feet. Come up onto the balls of your feet as you lift your feet very slightly off the floor. As you "skip", make a small circular motion with your hands, as if you were turning the rope. Repeat for a total of 32 skips.

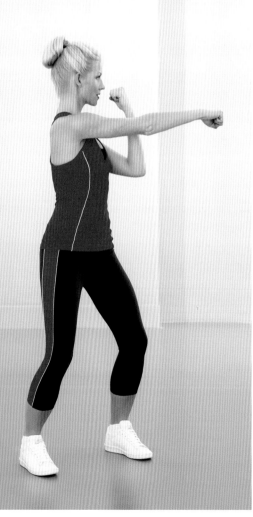

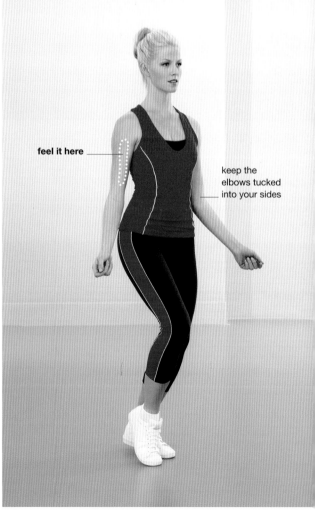

feel it here

keep the elbows tucked into your sides

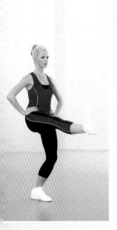

11 **Lunge kick** Starting with both feet together and hands on hips, kick one leg forward to hip-height, leading with the heel and flexing the foot. Return that leg behind to come into a lunge position resting on the toes. Repeat, making sure you keep your hips square and your knees always in line with your toes. Keep your tummy pulled in and your spine straight. Repeat for a total of 8 times, then change sides and repeat for a total of 8 times.

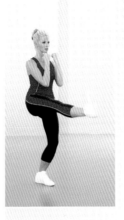

12 **Kick punch** Starting with your feet together and both hands held as fists under your chin, kick one leg forward to hip-height, leading with the heel and flexing the foot. As you return that leg behind you to rest it on its toes, punch the opposite arm across the body at chest-height. Repeat for a total of 8 times, then change sides and repeat for a total of 8 times. Repeat Step 10.

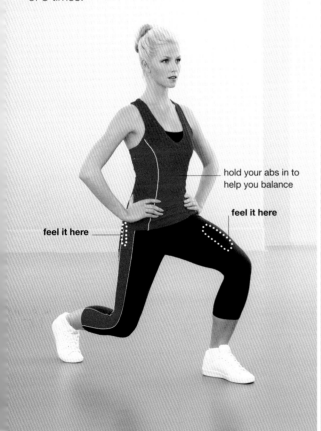

hold your abs in to help you balance

feel it here

feel it here

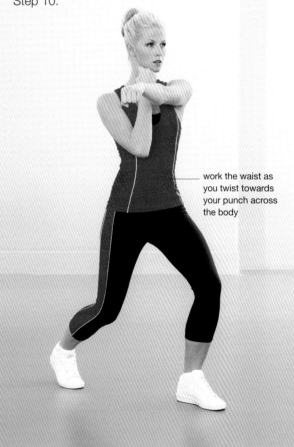

work the waist as you twist towards your punch across the body

13 **Ducks** Starting with your feet hip-width apart, hands in fists under your chin, squat down. Keep your weight in your heels. Straighten your knees and come to standing, leaning to one side with the opposite heel coming off the floor. Squat down again and lift up on the other side. Imagine you are ducking under a bar and coming up on alternate sides of it. Make sure you move through a full squat position before lifting up. Repeat for a total of 8 reps.

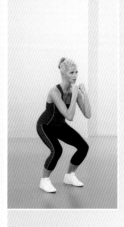

14 **Side-squat kick** Starting with your feet hip-width apart and both hands held as fists under your chin, squat down. Make sure your weight is in your heels. Then unbend your knees and come to standing, kicking out to the side with one leg. Lead with the heel and flex the foot. Repeat for a total of 4 times, returning to the centre squat position between each kick. Change sides and repeat for a total of 4 times. Repeat.

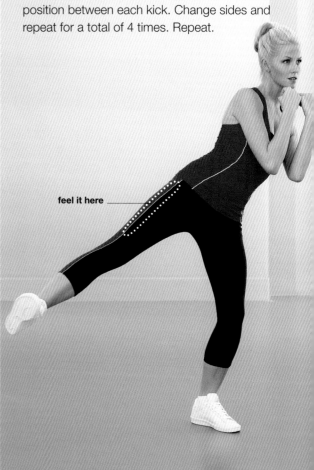

feel it here _____

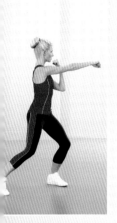

15 **Double-jab punch**
Starting with your
feet hip-width apart
and both hands held as fists
under your chin, double-
punch one arm across your
body at chest-height, keeping
the other fist under your chin.
First punch with the fist facing
the floor, then turn the arm
and punch upwards. Twist
your upper torso in the
direction of the punch, lifting
the opposite heel off the floor. Repeat on the
other side. Repeat for a total of 8 reps. Repeat
Step 10.

16 **Straight kick** Starting with your feet
together and both hands held as fists
under your chin, kick one leg forward
to hip-height, leading with the heel and flexing
the foot. Keep the supporting leg slightly bent,
and make sure the kicking foot returns parallel
to the supporting leg. Repeat for a total of 8
times, then change sides and repeat for a total
of 8 times. Repeat.

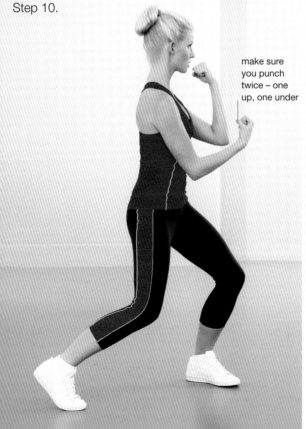

make sure
you punch
twice – one
up, one under

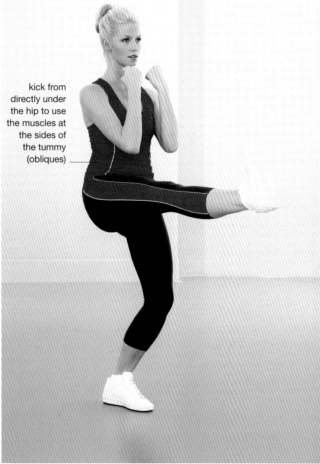

kick from
directly under
the hip to use
the muscles at
the sides of
the tummy
(obliques)

>> **workout** arm roll/bent-over twist

17 **Arm roll** Marching on the spot and with elbows at chest-height and shoulders relaxed, roll your forearms over each other in a circular motion. Roll them as fast as you can while you count to 16, then change direction for another count of 16.

18 **Bent-over twist** Take your feet wide and parallel, and with your knees slightly bent, bend at the waist to touch one hand to the outside of the opposite foot. As you touch, raise the other arm, keeping the elbow bent and pointing to the ceiling. Repeat, alternating sides, for a total of 16 reps.

Repeat Step 10, then Steps 9–12, then Step 10 again, then Steps 13–15, then Step 10 again, then Steps 16–18, and finally, Step 10 again.

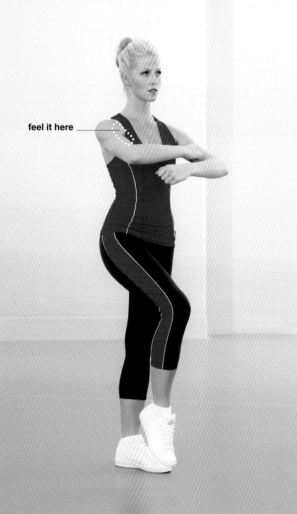

feel it here

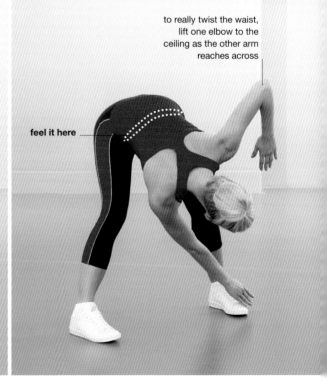

to really twist the waist, lift one elbow to the ceiling as the other arm reaches across

feel it here

19 **March** Standing on one foot, raise the other knee to hip-height. At the same time, raise the opposite arm. March on the spot, raising opposite knees and arms. Repeat for a total of 24 reps.

20 **Three-in-one stretch 1** Keeping both toes pointing forwards, take one leg behind you, and bend the front knee. Clasp your hands in front and raise your arms towards your ears as you lower your head. You should feel a stretch in your upper back, neck, and calf.

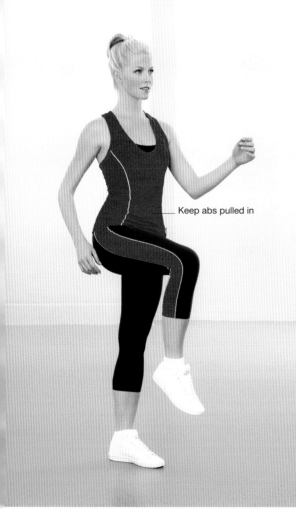

Keep abs pulled in

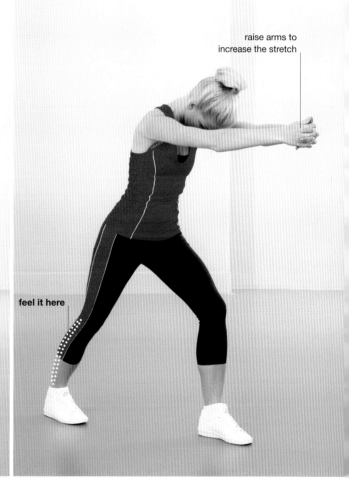

raise arms to increase the stretch

feel it here

>> **cool down** 3-in-1 stretch 2/quad stretch

21 **Three-in-one stretch 2** Take the other leg behind, toes pointing forward, and front knee bent. Clasp your hands behind your back. Open your chest as you raise your arms behind you. You should feel a stretch in your calf, chest, and arms.

22 **Quad stretch** Stand on one leg and hold the other foot with the hand on the same side. Bring the heel of the raised foot towards the buttock until you feel a stretch in the front of the bent-leg thigh. Change legs. If you cannot keep your balance, hold onto a support.

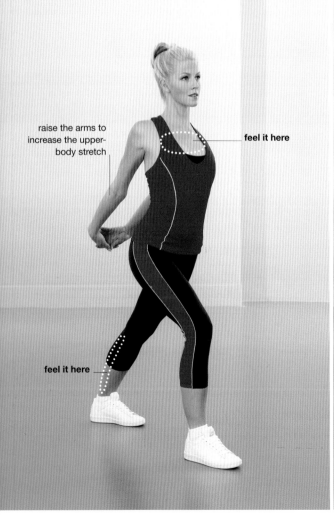

raise the arms to increase the upper-body stretch

feel it here

feel it here

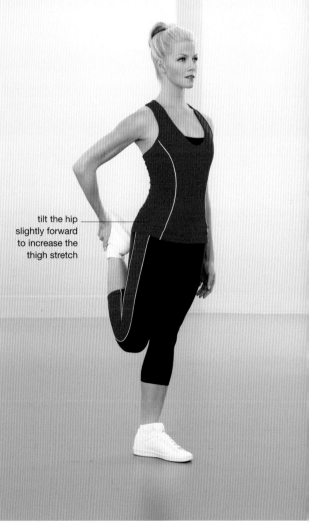

tilt the hip slightly forward to increase the thigh stretch

23 **Inner-thigh stretch** Take a step to one side and bend that knee, keeping the knee directly over the toes. Take your hands to the bent-leg thigh and lean forward, stretching the other leg out to the side. Make sure your neck and spine stay in line, and keep your back long and straight. You should feel a stretch in the inner thigh of the outstretched leg. Repeat on the other side.

24 **Roll-up** Stand tall with feet hip-width apart, arms stretched above your head, shoulders relaxed, and neck and spine in line. Slowly lower your arms and take your chin towards your chest, then round your back and slowly bend down towards the floor. When you are as low as possible, your hands should be relaxed and as near to the floor as is comfortable. Take a deep breath into your lower back. Then, keeping your tummy pulled into your lower back, uncurl slowly, one vertebra at a time, until you have returned to a standing position.

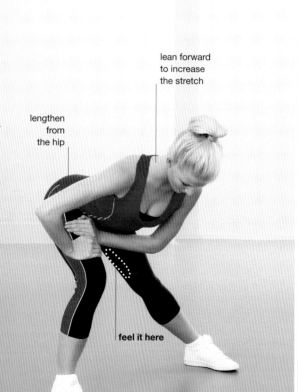

lean forward
to increase
the stretch

lengthen
from
the hip

feel it here

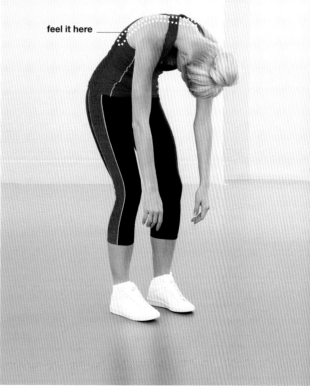

feel it here

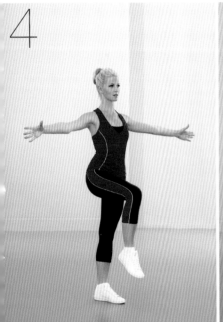

▲ **Warm up** March and flick,
page 23

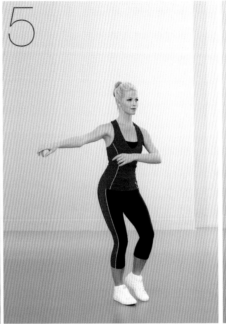

▲ **Warm up** Side step,
page 24

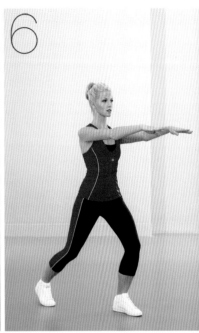

▲ **Warm up** Back step,
page 24

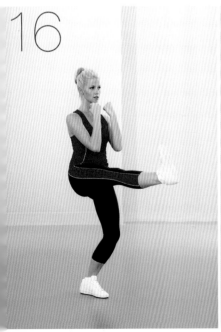

▲ **Workout** Straight kick,
page 29

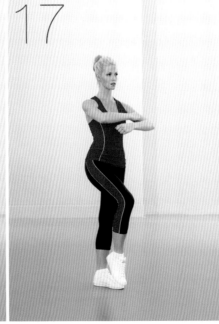

▲ **Workout** Arm roll,
page 30

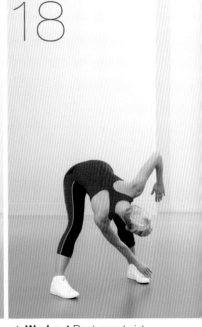

▲ **Workout** Bent-over twist,
page 30

boxing workout at a glance

1

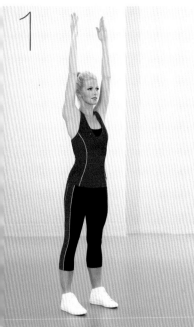

▲ **Warm up** Deep breaths,
page 22

2

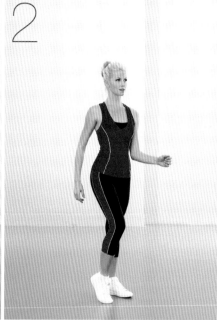

▲ **Warm up** Half-toe pump,
page 22

3

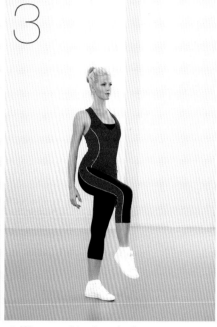

▲ **Warm up** March and roll,
page 23

13

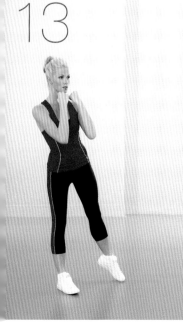

▲ **Workout** Ducks,
page 28

14

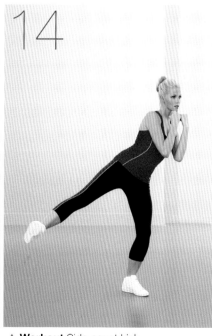

▲ **Workout** Side-squat kick,
page 28

15

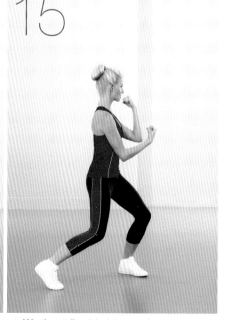

▲ **Workout** Double-jab punch,
page 29

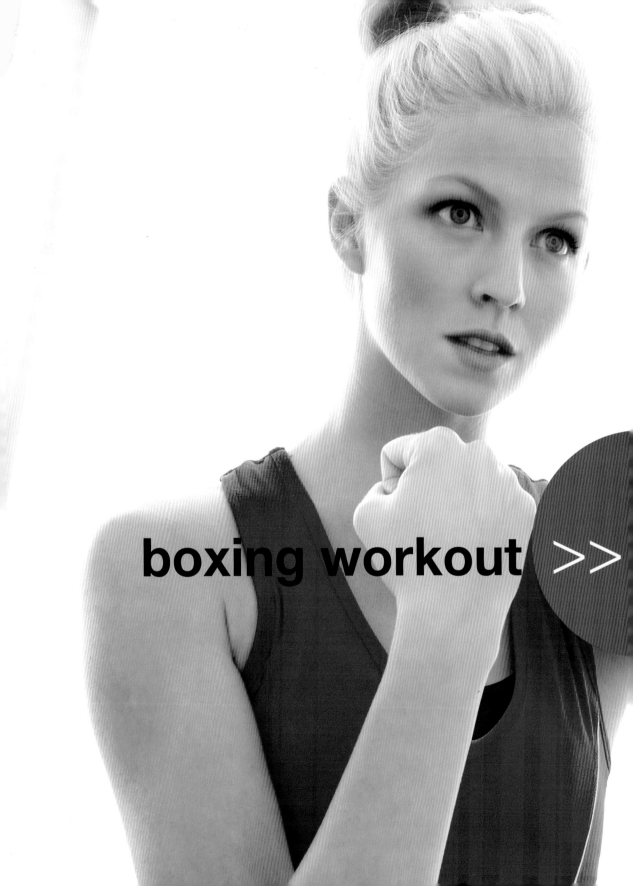

boxing workout >>

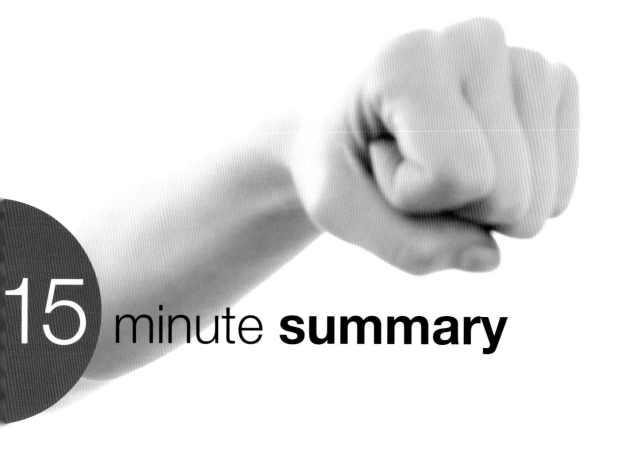

15 minute **summary**

10

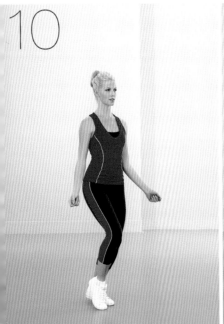

▲ **Workout** Skip,
page 26

11

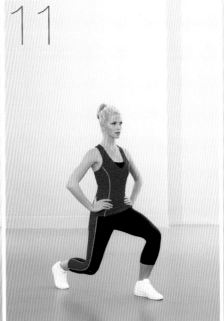

▲ **Workout** Lunge kick,
page 27

12

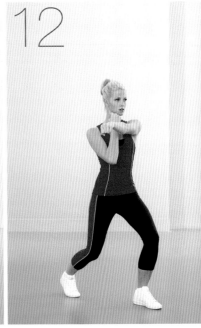

▲ **Workout** Kick punch,
page 27

22

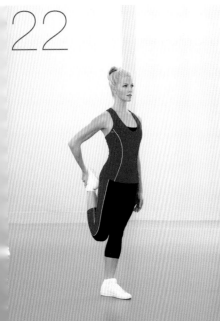

▲ **Cool down** Quad stretch,
page 32

23

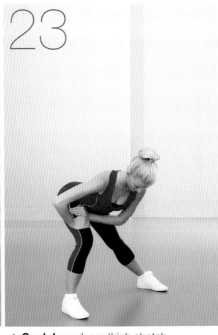

▲ **Cool down** Inner-thigh stretch,
page 33

24

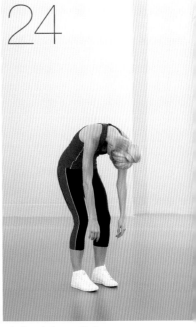

▲ **Cool down** Roll-up,
page 33

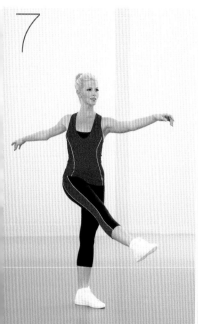

7

▲ **Warm up** Dip-kick with twist, page 25

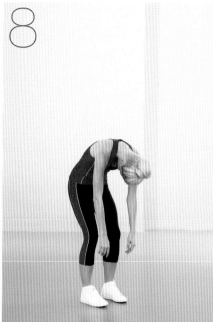

8

▲ **Warm up** Roll-up, page 25

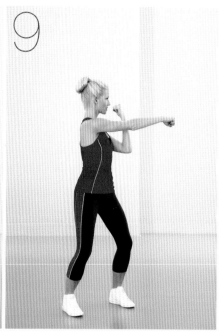

9

▲ **Workout** Punch across, page 26

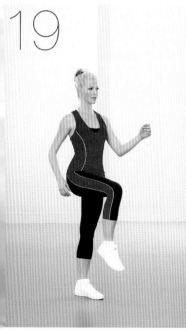

19

▲ **Cool down** March, page 31

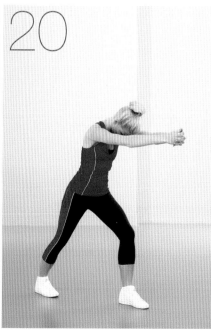

20

▲ **Cool down** 3-in-1 stretch 1, page 31

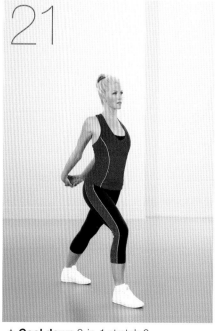

21

▲ **Cool down** 3-in-1 stretch 2, page 32

>> **boxing workout** FAQs

Challenging and intense, this workout will get the most into, and out of, your 15 minutes. Keep your abs pulled up, particularly with the kicks in this sequence. That work, plus the upper-body punching and arm rolls, really makes this an all-round toner and calorie-buster.

>> I find the ducking movement in Ducks awkward, and can't seem to get down and up in time. How can I get the hang of it?

Imagine you are ducking under and popping up on either side of a bar or rope. Your lower body stays firm, and you are leaning slightly from the waist as you come up. If you can't get up in time, try not bending your knees so much. Instead, concentrate on the leaning to the side from the waist. It will give you a good waist trim!

>> I seem to be a few steps behind when I'm following the DVD. How can I improve?

This is the first sequence in the book, so chances are it's the first one you're attempting. You'll improve the more you do this or any of the sequences. Just remember that to burn calories the important thing is to keep moving! If there's a particular point that always trips you up, check the picture instruction on the relevant page, and practise the move or transition a few times.

>> I can't keep my balance kicking out to the side in the Side-squat kick. What am I doing wrong?

Make sure you keep your weight centred. Holding your tummy in helps. The leg you are standing on should always be slightly bent, and when you bend both knees they should always be facing forward and in line with the toes. When you kick to the side, think of leading with your heel, not your hip.

>> **I feel stiff and tight in my neck and shoulders when I'm doing this workout, and sometimes afterwards. Is that normal?**

It is very important to relax your neck and shoulders whatever exercise you are doing, and as there are so many arm and upper body moves here, you have to be on guard. You will notice that when you make a fist with your hand (as you do when you are punching) the tension tends to work up to your neck. Don't let it! Practise making a fist and relaxing your neck at the same time. Also be aware when you have your hands in the "guard" position (fists under your chin) that you don't use your shoulders to keep them there. Finally, make sure you do the neck and upper back stretch thoroughly in the cool-down.

>> **How high do I need to kick my leg in the Lunge kick, the Kick punch, the Side-squat kick, and the Straight kick?**

Some of the kicking moves warrant a higher finish than the others. For example, the Lunge kick should have you kicking higher than the Kick punch, the Side-squat kick or the Straight kick. In general, you should go as high as you can without compromising your posture or form. If your standing leg is being lifted or pulled out of position when you kick the other leg, and/or you are unsteady, then you're kicking too high.

>> **I feel a "burning" sensation in the front of my thighs, especially when I'm doing the kicking movements. What am I doing wrong?**

If you feel "burning" in your thighs, it means your quads are doing all the work. Try to work from your centre, that's to say your tummy, and think of lifting your leg from there, instead of from the top of your thigh. Focus your effort into your abdominal area by keeping your tummy pulled in, your back nice and straight, and your standing leg very slightly bent.

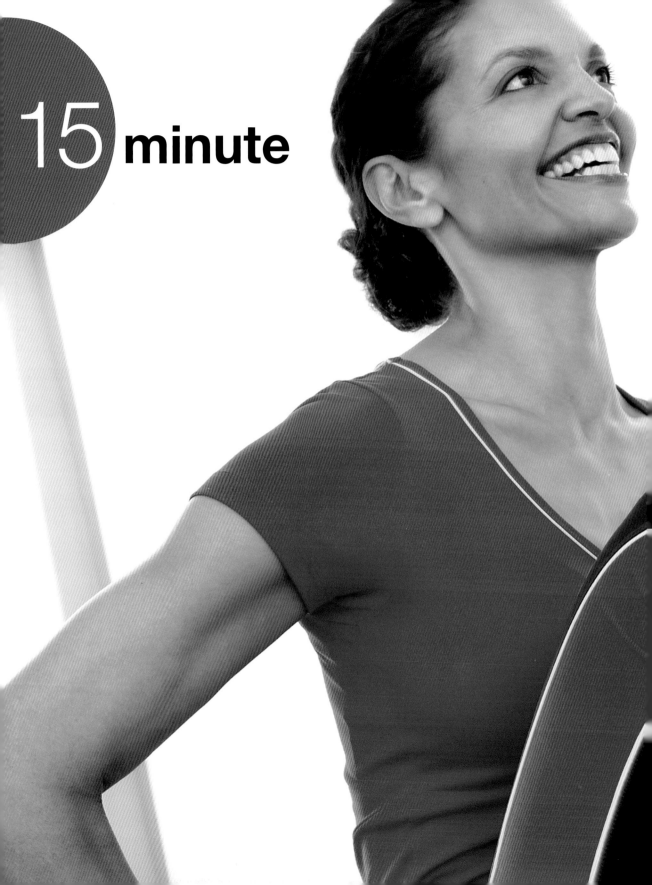

15 minute

aerobic
workout >>

Step, march, hop, jump! Raise your heart rate and your spirit as you exercise the old school way!

>> **aerobic** workout

Think of an aerobics workout and the chances are you'll conjure up an image of a class involving women wearing headbands and a lot of Lycra. That's how things were in the 1980s. This sequence offers you my collection of classic aerobic moves. Headbands and Lycra are optional!

The term "aerobics" was first used to describe a system of exercise which an exercise physiologist designed to help prevent heart disease. The system involved doing continuous, rhythmic activity using large muscle groups. In fact, all the sequences in my *15 Minute Calorie Burn Workout* are "aerobic", which is why they help you to burn calories.

The aerobics classes most of us recognize today have evolved from what started out in the US in the early 1970s and grew into a worldwide craze that became one of the defining features of the 1980s. If you happened to be around then – as I was – you may recall the hype that surrounded particular classes. The combination of exercise, music, and the social aspect often proved irresistible. And because you could – and still can – work more or less intensively, depending on your ability, one of the advantages of aerobics classes was that they gave people of different fitness levels the chance to work together and have fun.

My own Aerobic Workout offers you the chance to do a collection of some classic – what I would call "vintage" – aerobic steps from the early days. Some of the moves, such as the Grapevine, Toe tap, and Rocking horse, were around then, and are often to be found in classes today.

Many of the steps in this aerobic workout are very simple, so it is important to monitor how hard you are training. Ideally, you should aim to work at a level where you are not too comfortable. If the steps feel easy to you, follow the tips on pp16–17 to intensify your work rate. However, some of the

> ## >> **tips for** my aerobic workout
>
> - **In Chest march,** you have to really relax the shoulders and arms to isolate the chest muscles properly. Your elbows should meet (or nearly meet) as you flex the chest.
>
> - **In Side-dig swing,** don't transfer all your weight to the foot you step out on. Keep your weight centred and "bounce" the step more. This helps you to keep in time.
>
> - **In high-impact steps** such as Crossover jump, be sure to land correctly, flexing your knees and rolling through your feet. Do it safely and don't rush it.

steps – for example, Chest march, Side-dig swing, and Crossover jump – need your special attention (see above). And remember: quality is always more important than quantity.

Although you will be doing this workout in the comfort of your own home, imagine yourself in a 1980s class. Let yourself go and have fun. Perform the moves with enthusiasm. You could even get the rest of your family involved!

One of the benefits of doing a regular aerobics workout is that you can perform the steps with an intensity that suits you, and still burn up the calories.

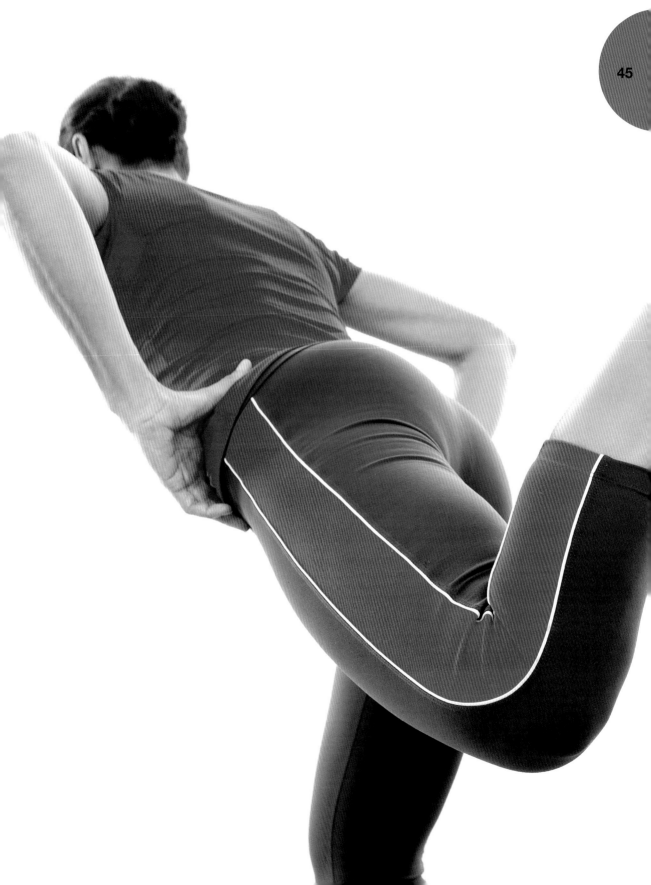

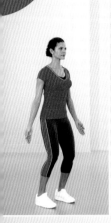

>> **warm up** deep breaths/half-toe pump

1 **Deep breaths** Stand tall with feet hip-width apart, knees soft, and arms by your sides. Relax your neck and shoulders, and make sure your tummy is pulled in. Take a deep breath in as you bend the knees and raise your arms above your head. Exhale as you lower them with a smooth circular movement. Make sure your back stays straight. Repeat for a total of 4 reps.

to really lengthen your spine, lift from the hips as you raise the arms upwards

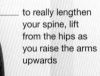

2 **Half-toe pump** Alternate your weight from one foot to the other, rising up onto the ball of your foot. As you alternate feet, curl the opposite arm to your shoulder. Keep your hands in a loose fist and make sure you push your heel right down to the floor as you work your calf muscle. Repeat for a total of 16 reps (1 rep = both sides/directions).

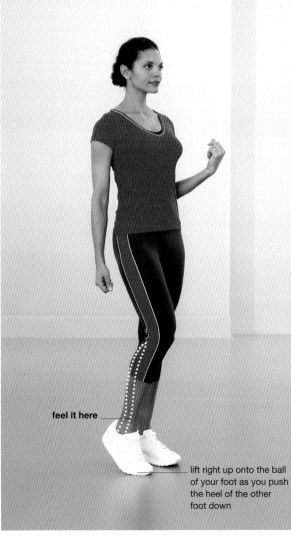

feel it here

lift right up onto the ball of your foot as you push the heel of the other foot down

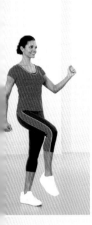

3 **March and roll** Standing on one foot, raise the other knee to waist-height. At the same time, raise the opposite arm. March on the spot, raising opposite knees and arms. Repeat for a total of 8 reps. Then, with your arms by your sides, raise your shoulders towards your ears and roll them in a circular motion, backwards, then forwards. Repeat for a total of 4 reps.

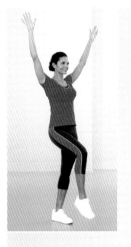

4 **March and flick** Continue marching and, as you do so, stretch your arms sideways to meet above your head, opening and closing your hands at intervals with a "flicking" motion, to warm your fingers and wrists. Continue "flicking" your hands as you lower your arms. Repeat for a total of 4 reps.

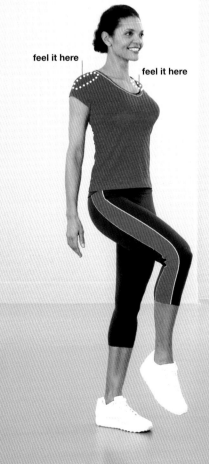

feel it here

feel it here

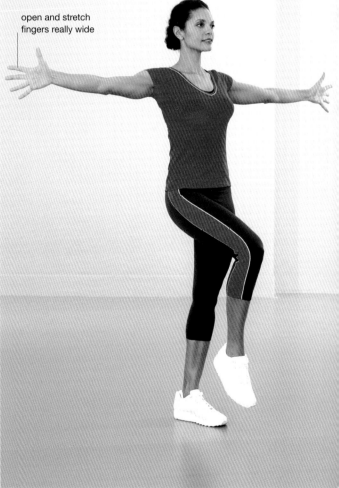

open and stretch fingers really wide

>> **warm up** side step/back step

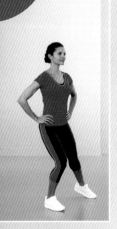

5 **Side step** With hands on hips, take a step to one side, then bring your feet together. Repeat to the other side. Repeat for a total of 4 reps, then swing your arms in the same direction as you are stepping. Your arms should be relaxed and raised no higher than shoulder-height. Repeat for a total of 8 reps.

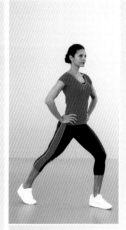

6 **Back step** With hands on hips, touch one foot on the floor behind you. Return to centre. Repeat with the opposite foot. Keep your weight centred as you alternate legs. Repeat for a total of 4 reps, then add an arm push in time with your leg movements by pushing both arms forward and back just below shoulder-height. Repeat for a total of 8 reps.

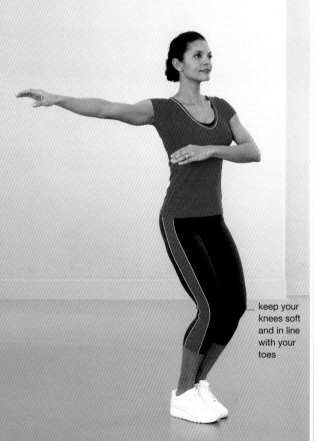

keep your knees soft and in line with your toes

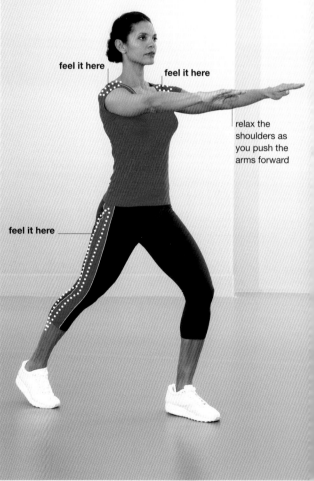

feel it here

feel it here

relax the shoulders as you push the arms forward

feel it here

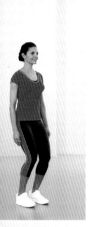

7 **Dip-kick with twist** With arms by your sides, bend both knees, then come up and kick one foot forward. Repeat for a total of 8 reps, then add a twist by turning your upper body and swinging the opposite arm to the kicking leg. Keep the arms shoulder-height. Keep your hips square. Repeat, alternating sides, for a total of 8 reps.

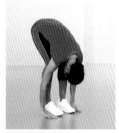

8 **Roll-up** Stand tall with feet hip-width apart, arms stretched above your head, shoulders relaxed, and neck and spine in line. Slowly lower your arms and take your chin towards your chest, then round your back and slowly bend down towards the floor. When you are as low as possible, your hands should be relaxed and as near to the floor as is comfortable. Take a deep breath into your lower back. Then, keeping your tummy pulled into your lower back, uncurl slowly, one vertebra at a time, until you have returned to a standing position.

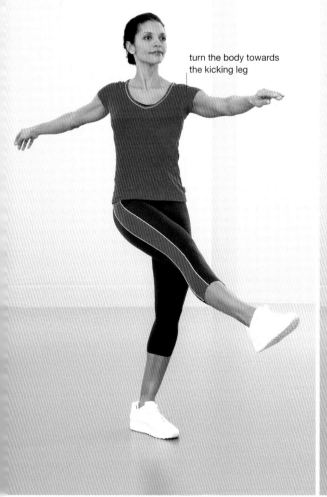

turn the body towards the kicking leg

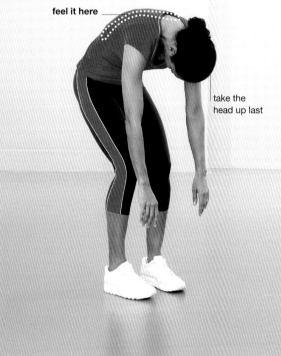

feel it here

take the head up last

>> **workout** toe tap/march

9 **Toe tap** Standing with feet apart and knees slightly turned out, tap the toes of one foot on the floor to the side. As you tap, curl your arms at the elbow, alternating arms. Repeat for a total of 16 reps, then change feet and repeat for a total of 16 reps.

10 **March** Standing on one foot, raise the other knee to waist-height. At same time, raise the opposite arm. March on the spot, raising opposite knees and arms. Repeat for a total of 16 reps.

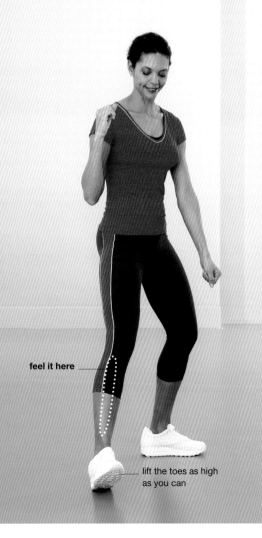

feel it here

lift the toes as high as you can

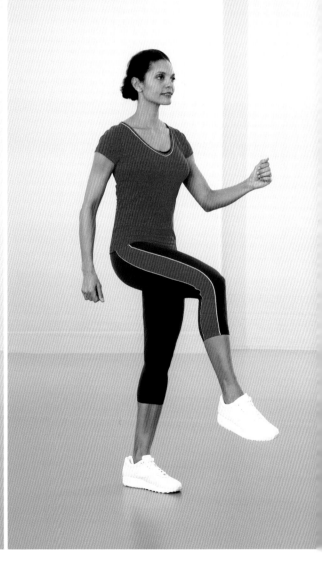

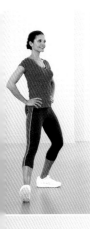

11 **Grapevine** With hands on hips, step to the side, take the other foot behind, step to the side again, then bring the feet together. Repeat on the other side. Repeat for a total of 4 reps.

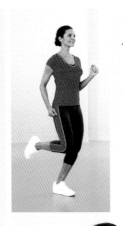

12 **Jump-kick punch** Starting with both feet together, hop onto one leg, bend the other, then kick that leg forward. As you kick, raise the opposite arm skywards and keep the arm on the same side behind and slightly bent at the elbow. Repeat, alternating sides, for a total of 8 reps. Repeat Step 11.

punch forward with palm side of the fist down

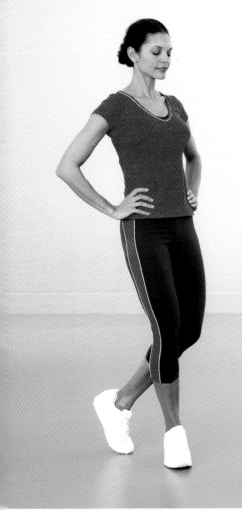

>> **workout** crossover jump/chest march

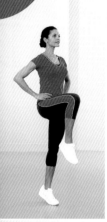

13 **Crossover jump**
Starting with both feet together and hands on hips, jump, taking one knee to hip-height. Cross that leg over the other, touching the toe briefly to the floor. Bring the knee back to hip-height, then back to centre. Repeat on the other side. Repeat for a total of 8 reps.

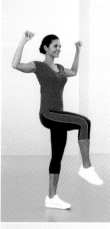

14 **Chest march**
Standing on one foot, raise the other knee to hip-height and take the arms to the sides at shoulder-height, elbows bent. March on the spot, bringing the elbows together at chest-height, then opening them. Repeat for a total of 16 times.

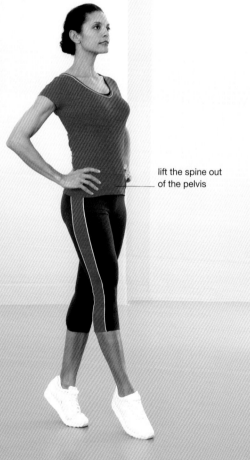

lift the spine out of the pelvis

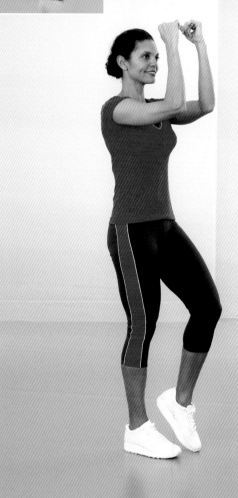

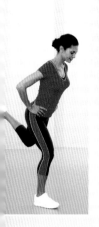

15 **Rocking horse** Starting with both feet together and hands on hips, step forward onto one foot and bend the other leg behind at the knee. Rock slightly onto the front leg. Step the back leg down, raise the front leg and rock slightly onto the back leg. Repeat the forward and back rocking motion for a total of 8 reps. Change sides and repeat for a total of 8 reps. Repeat Step 11.

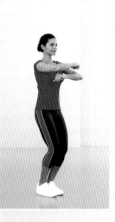

16 **Side-dig swing** Starting with both feet together and arms in front of you at chest-height with elbows bent, step to one side. As you step, open the arms to the sides, elbows still bent. Bring the feet and arms together, then step to the other side and open the arms again. Repeat, alternating sides, for a total of 8 reps.

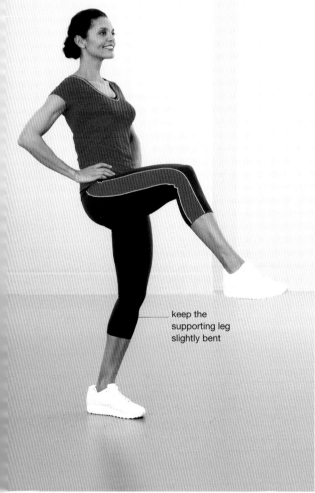

keep the supporting leg slightly bent

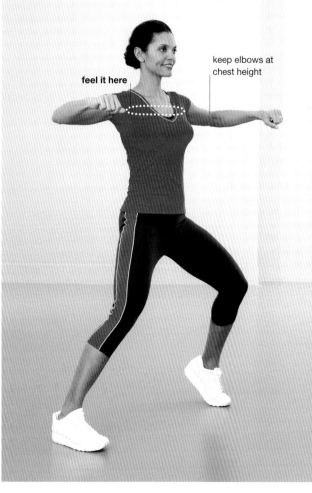

feel it here

keep elbows at chest height

>> **workout** jog/cross-country ski

17 **Jog** Curling the opposite arm to the lifted knee, jog on the spot, raising your heels towards your buttocks. Make sure your heels touch the ground every time you land. Repeat for a total of 16 reps.

18 **Cross-country ski** Standing on one leg, take the arm on the same side up and forward and take the other leg behind. The other arm stays by your side. Keeping the knees bent, change sides. Repeat, alternating sides, for a total of 4 reps. Make sure you work from your centre, keeping your tummy pulled in for good balance.

Repeat Step 11, then Steps 9–12, then Step 11 again, then Steps 13–15, then Step 11 again, then Steps 16–18, then Step 11 again, then Steps 9–12, then Step 11 again, then Steps 13–15, then Step 11 again, then Steps 16–18, and finally, Step 11 again.

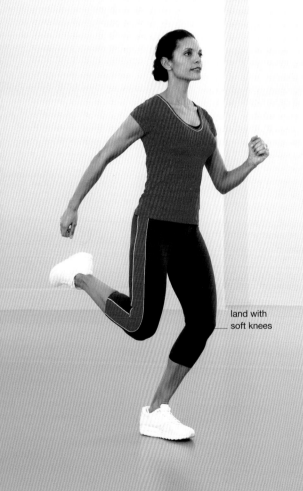

land with
soft knees

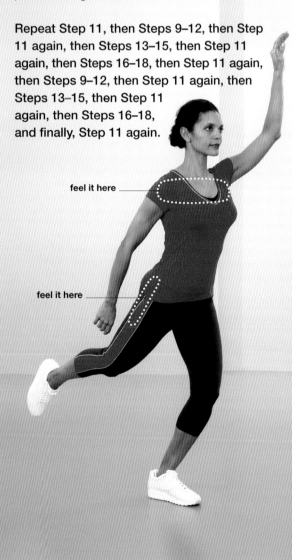

feel it here

feel it here

19 **March** Standing on one foot, raise the other knee to hip-height. At the same time, raise the opposite arm. March on the spot, raising opposite knees and arms. Repeat for a total of 24 reps.

20 **Three-in-one stretch 1** Keeping both toes pointing forward, take one leg behind you, and bend the front knee. Clasp your hands in front and raise your arms towards your ears as you lower your head. You should feel a stretch in your upper back, neck, and calf.

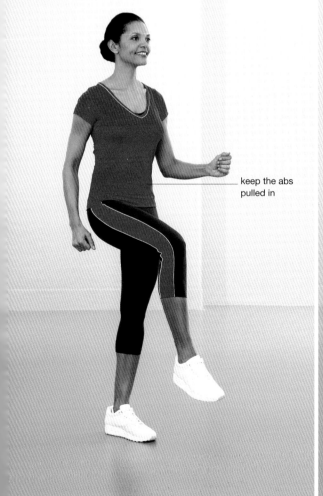

keep the abs
pulled in

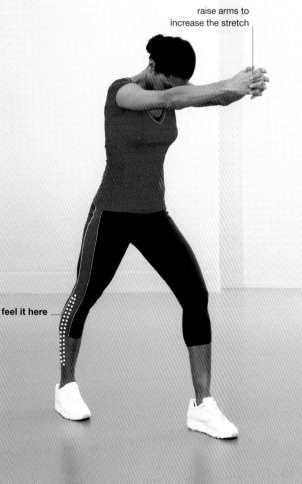

raise arms to
increase the stretch

feel it here

>> **cool down** 3-in-1 stretch 2/quad stretch

21 **Three-in-one stretch 2** Take the other leg behind, toes pointing forward, and front knee bent. Clasp your hands behind your back. Open your chest as you raise your arms behind you. You should feel a stretch in your calf, chest, and arms.

22 **Quad stretch** Stand on one leg and hold the other foot with the hand on the same side. Bring the heel of the raised foot towards the buttock until you feel a stretch in the front of the bent-leg thigh. Change legs. If you cannot keep your balance, hold onto a support.

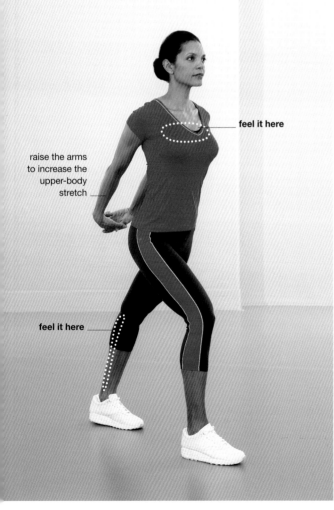

feel it here

raise the arms to increase the upper-body stretch

feel it here

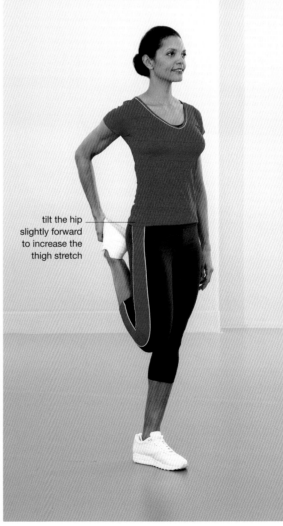

tilt the hip slightly forward to increase the thigh stretch

23 **Inner-thigh stretch** Take a step to one side and bend that knee, keeping the knee directly over the toes. Take your hands to the bent-leg thigh and lean forward, stretching the other leg out to the side. Make sure your neck and spine stay in line, and keep your back long and straight. You should feel a stretch in the inner thigh of the outstretched leg. Repeat on the other side.

24 **Roll-up** Stand tall with feet hip-width apart, arms stretched above your head, shoulders relaxed, and neck and spine in line. Slowly lower your arms and take your chin towards your chest, then round your back and slowly bend down towards the floor. When you are as low as possible, your hands should be relaxed and as near to the floor as is comfortable. Take a deep breath into your lower back. Then, keeping your tummy pulled into your lower back, uncurl slowly, one vertebra at a time, until you have returned to a standing position.

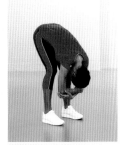

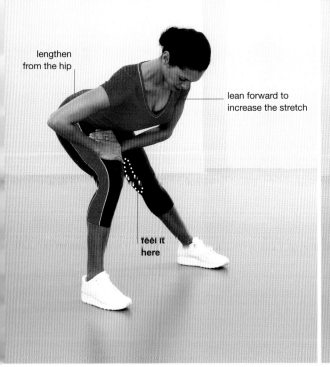

lengthen from the hip

lean forward to increase the stretch

feel it here

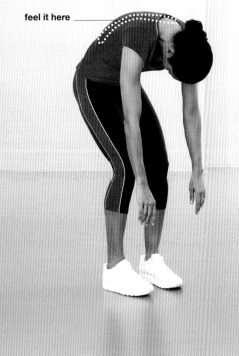

feel it here

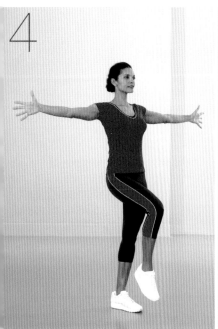

▲ **Warm up** March and flick,
page 47

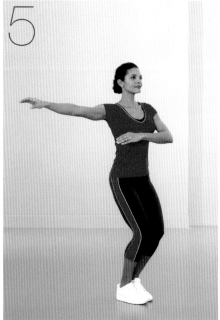

▲ **Warm up** Side step,
page 48

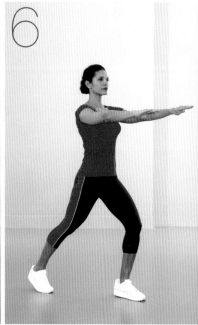

▲ **Warm up** Back step,
page 48

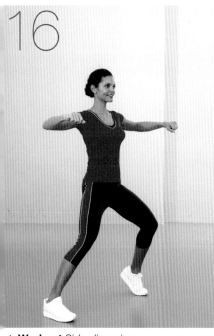

▲ **Workout** Side-dig swing,
page 53

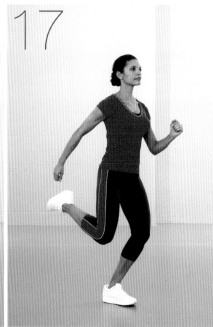

▲ **Workout** Jog,
page 54

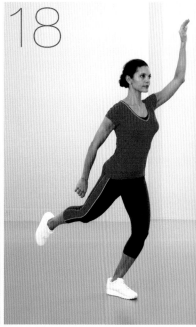

▲ **Workout** Cross-country ski,
page 54

aerobic workout at a glance

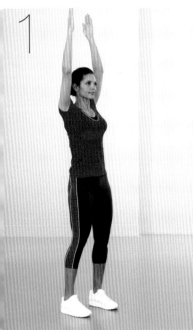

▲ **Warm up** Deep breaths,
page 46

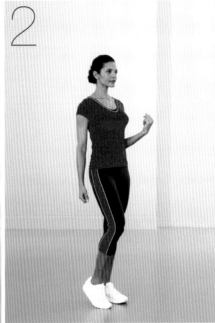

▲ **Warm up** Half-toe pump,
page 46

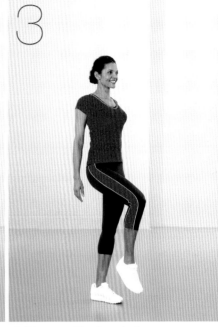

▲ **Warm up** March and roll,
page 47

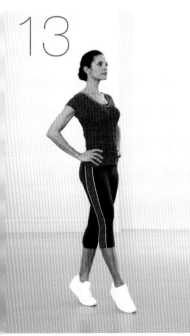

▲ **Workout** Crossover jump,
page 52

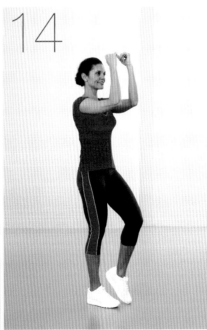

▲ **Workout** Chest march,
page 52

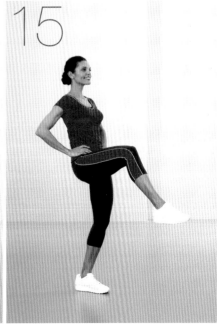

▲ **Workout** Rocking horse,
page 53

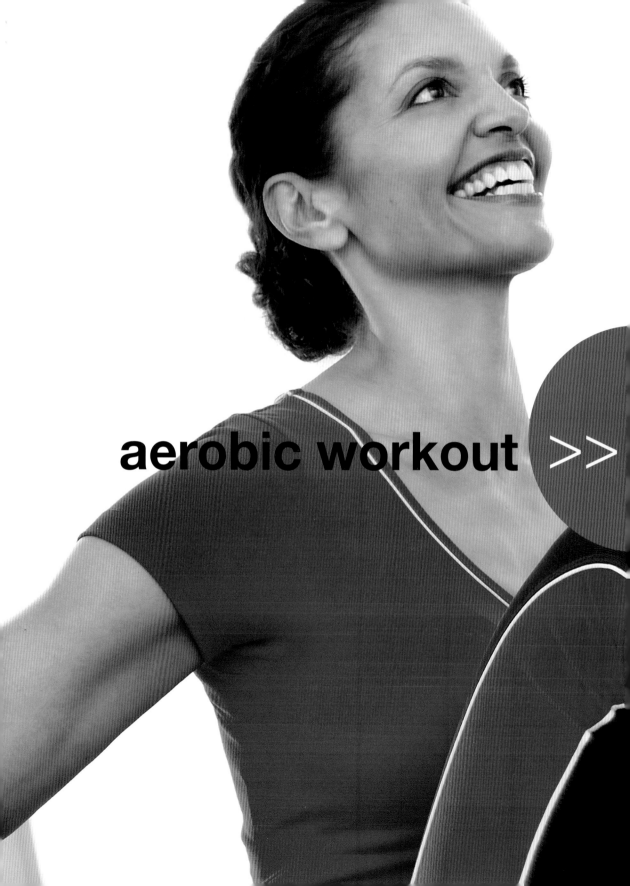

aerobic workout >>

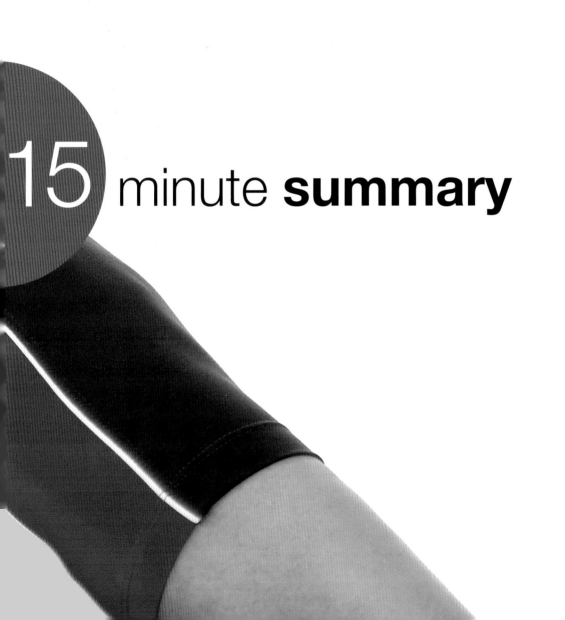

15 minute **summary**

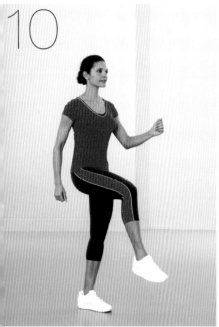

10

▲ **Workout** March,
page 50

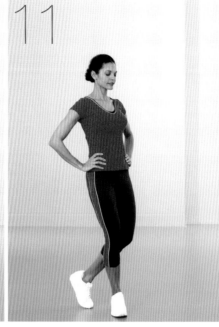

11

▲ **Workout** Grapevine,
page 51

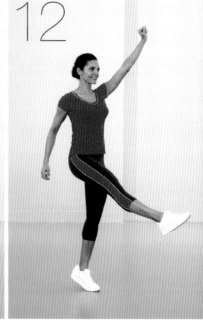

12

▲ **Workout** Jump-kick punch,
page 51

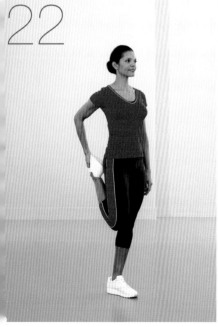

22

▲ **Cool down** Quad stretch,
page 56

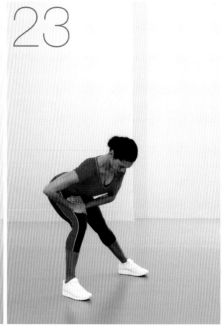

23

▲ **Cool down** Inner-thigh stretch,
page 57

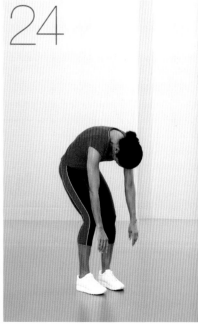

24

▲ **Cool down** Roll-up,
page 57

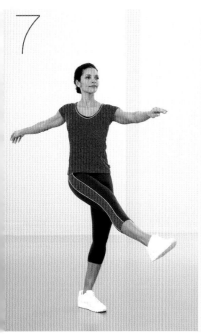

▲ **Warm up** Dip-kick with twist,
page 49

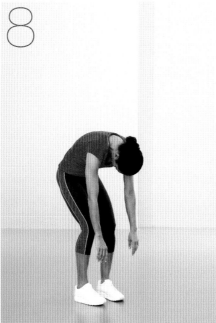

▲ **Warm up** Roll-up,
page 49

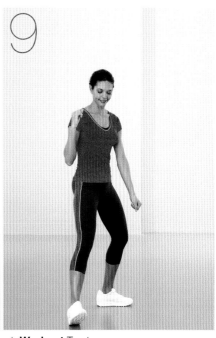

▲ **Workout** Toe tap,
page 50

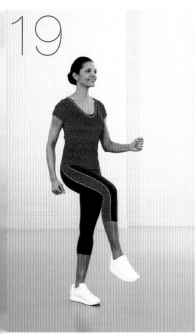

▲ **Cool down** March,
page 55

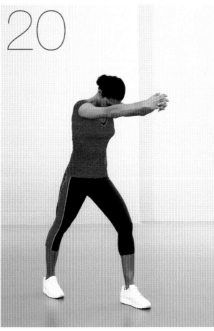

▲ **Cool down** 3-in-1 stretch 1,
page 55

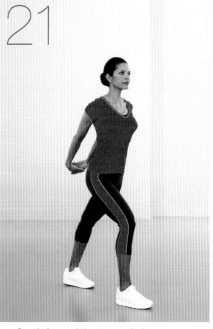

▲ **Cool down** 3-in-1 stretch 2,
page 56

>> **aerobic workout** FAQs

Aerobics classes are probably the best known of all exercise classes and chances are you have taken part in or at least seen an aerobics class. This workout is a great all-rounder as you are working on your heart and lungs, as well as on your coordination and muscle toning.

>> **I find the Crossover jump difficult. Is there some way I can simplify it?**

This is a real high-impact step, and involves jumping as you lift the knee up, as well as when you cross it over. If you cannot seem to get all the moves in within the timing, do a low-impact version instead – lifting the knee up and over without the jump.

>> **What if I don't have enough space to really travel the Grapevine?**

If you cannot take your steps wide, make this move work by exaggerating the bend in your knees as you cross the leg behind, and exaggerating it again as you join the feet together at the end of each step. This creates more depth and will compensate calorie-wise for taking smaller steps.

>> **Can I do anything with my arms when I do the Grapevine, instead of always having my hands on my hips?**

The Grapevine is an absolute classic and has endless variations. Once you're confident about your footwork, you can add any arm movements that feel good. My favourite is pushing my arms up towards the ceiling and slightly out to the sides (ten to three and ten past three) in time with my steps. And you can always add a hand clap as your feet come together for that classic Eighties feel!

>> **I don't feel as if anything is happening when doing the Toe tap. Am I doing something wrong in this move?**

You will be surprised how much you can push this little step! Really lift the toes while your heel stays firmly planted. As you lift your flexed foot, you should feel not only your shins, but your calf muscle as well.

>> **I don't know what I'm supposed to be working when I do the Cross-country ski. Can you explain what is going on?**

This is a great exercise for your abdominals and lower back (core) as well as for the back of your legs (hamstrings) and your upper back. Make sure your supporting leg is bent enough so you can lean forward, and keep your abs pulled in to help you keep your balance. If you want to intensify the move, exaggerate the lean forward and really squeeze your butt as you lift the leg behind. As you lower your arm, focus on the muscles in your chest.

>> **My legs, and especially my thighs, feel particularly tired when I'm doing this workout. Am I doing something wrong?**

Classic aerobics steps, which is what this sequence is built on, are based on the lower body. When you are using the larger muscle groups of this part of the body – those of the legs and the buttocks – you work harder, which is why these are usually the focus of any aerobic workout. During your Cool Down, concentrate on the Quad stretch (see p56) to stretch out the quads (fronts of the thighs) after you've completed the sequence. And remember, if you have any burning or cramping sensation that you cannot work through, it is fine to pause for 15–20 seconds and stretch out one or both thighs.

15 minute

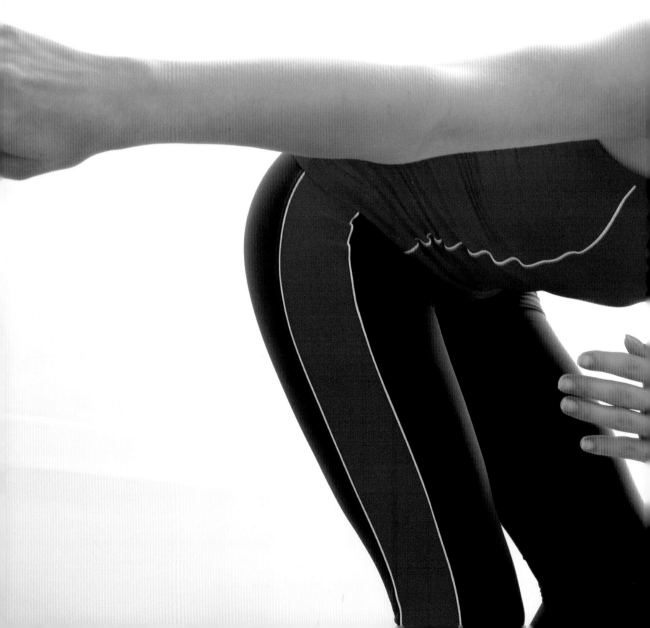

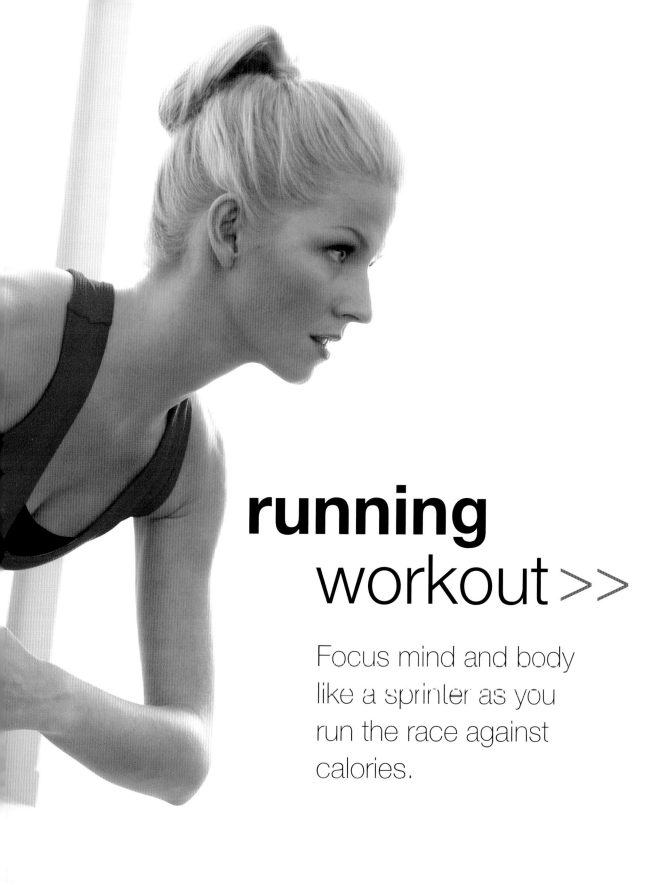

running
workout >>

Focus mind and body like a sprinter as you run the race against calories.

>> **running** workout

Running or jogging outside, especially through a park or on a sandy beach, can't be beaten. Unfortunately, we don't all have those locations on our doorstep, nor an hour or more to spare. So unless you've got a treadmill in your living room, this sequence is the next best thing!

Running is great for your heart and cardiovascular system, and for burning calories, which is why I have included running in this programme. This particular sequence, which incorporates jogging and some sprint-training exercises, is one of the more vigorous workouts in the book. While you are doing it, you'll not only be working out as intensely as you would if you were running outdoors, but you'll also be toning and shaping your muscles.

The downside of running, though, is that your knees and hips undergo a good deal of sustained impact. And for women, there is also the problem of proper bust support. So, before you begin, invest in a good pair of trainers and a sports bra (see pp14–15), even if you don't have a big bust.

To keep this Running Workout as intense as possible and to burn the maximum calories, try to maintain your level of effort throughout. Don't think of the March as less demanding than the Jog, or as an opportunity for a bit of a break. If you really want to burn calories, put ideas like that out of your mind and keep working at a good rate by raising your knees high and really swinging your arms through.

You may think the Step pump is also a good time to catch your breath. Again, if you really want to burn calories, you should intensify your work by exaggerating the contrast between the crouching forward movement and coming back up to standing.

Although the Lunges are performed more slowly than the other steps in the sequence, they are still not an opportunity to take it easy. Lunges are always very taxing, and even more so when you

> ## >> **tips for** my running workout
>
> - **Whenever you land** – for instance, after a hop or a jump – aim for a soft landing with minimum impact. This means keeping your knees soft and rolling through your whole foot, not just landing on your toes.
>
> - **In the Sprint start,** mimic a sprinter at the start of a race. Really power from low to high as you raise your knees towards your chest.
>
> - **In Ski runs,** stay low to the ground, take big steps, and move as far forwards and back as you can. In a small space, bend the knees to increase the depth of movement.

have to slow them right down as you do here. To burn those calories, make sure you follow all the tips to get your technique totally perfect and use the concept of "mind to muscle" (see p16) to help you focus on exactly which parts of your body you are working. Lunges don't just work your thighs. The backs of your legs and your bottom should be working hard, too, so focus your weight into your heels. That will help to remind them to work!

When you're performing this sequence, work your limbs at a good consistent rate and keep your shoulders and neck relaxed as you swing your arms through.

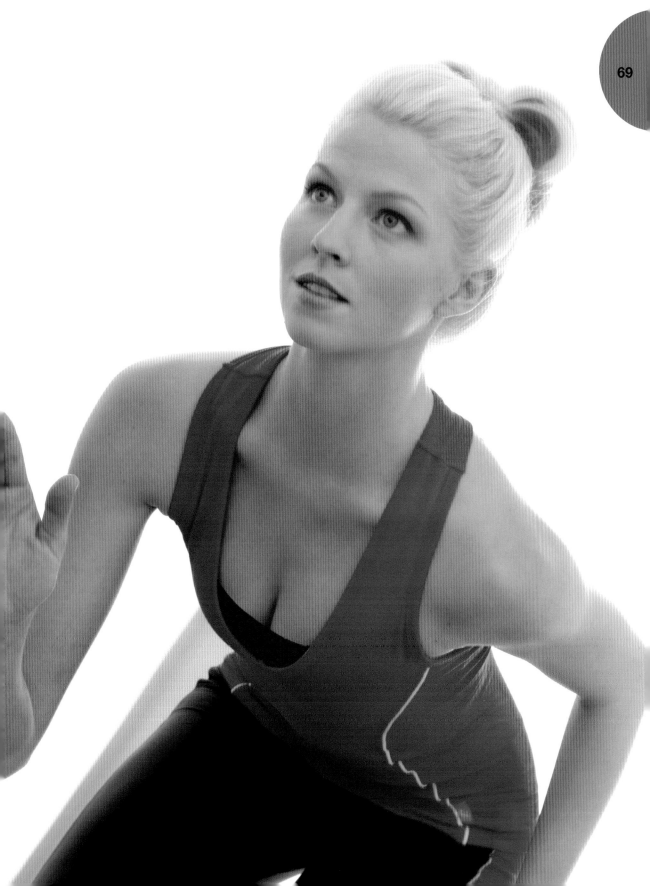

>> **warm up** deep breaths/half-toe pump

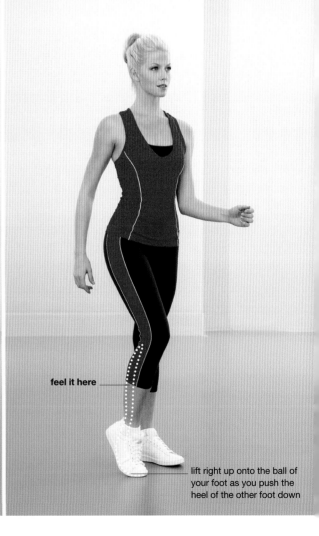

1 **Deep breaths** Stand tall with feet hip-width apart, knees soft, and arms by your sides. Relax your neck and shoulders, and make sure your tummy is pulled in. Take a deep breath in as you bend the knees and raise your arms above your head. Exhale as you lower them with a smooth circular movement. Make sure your back stays straight. Repeat for a total of 4 reps.

2 **Half-toe pump** Alternate your weight from one foot to the other, rising up onto the ball of your foot. As you alternate feet, curl the opposite arm to your shoulder. Keep your hands in a loose fist and make sure you push your heel right down to the floor as you work your calf muscle. Repeat for a total of 16 reps (1 rep = both sides/directions).

to really lengthen your spine, lift from the hips as you raise the arms upwards

feel it here

lift right up onto the ball of your foot as you push the heel of the other foot down

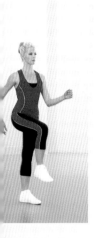

3 **March and roll** Standing on one foot, raise the other knee to waist-height. At the same time, raise the opposite arm. March on the spot, raising opposite knees and arms. Repeat for a total of 8 reps. Then, with your arms by your sides, raise your shoulders towards your ears and roll them in a circular motion, backwards, then forwards. Repeat for a total of 4 reps.

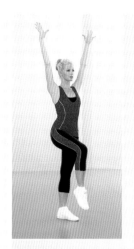

4 **March and flick** Continue marching and, as you do so, stretch your arms sideways to meet above your head, opening and closing your hands at intervals with a "flicking" motion, to warm your fingers and wrists. Continue "flicking" your hands as you lower your arms. Repeat for a total of 4 reps.

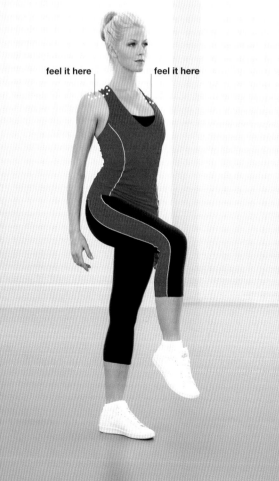

feel it here   feel it here

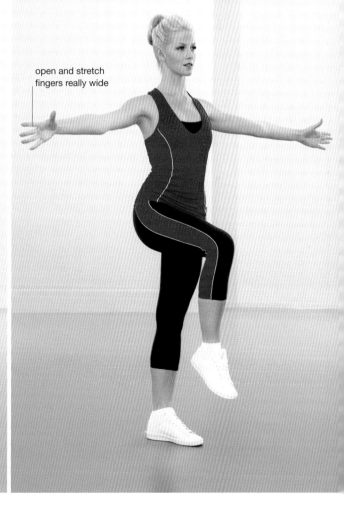

open and stretch fingers really wide

>> **warm up** side step/back step

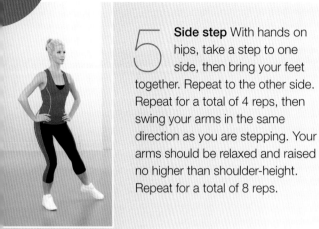

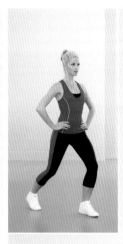

5 **Side step** With hands on hips, take a step to one side, then bring your feet together. Repeat to the other side. Repeat for a total of 4 reps, then swing your arms in the same direction as you are stepping. Your arms should be relaxed and raised no higher than shoulder-height. Repeat for a total of 8 reps.

6 **Back step** With hands on hips, touch one foot on the floor behind you. Return to centre and repeat with the opposite foot. Keep your weight centred as you alternate legs. Repeat for a total of 4 reps, then add an arm push in time with your leg movements by pushing both arms forward and back just below shoulder-height. Repeat for a total of 8 reps.

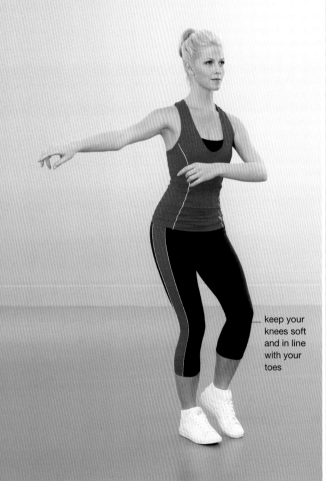

keep your knees soft and in line with your toes

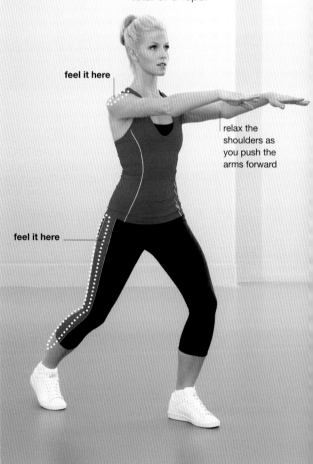

feel it here

relax the shoulders as you push the arms forward

feel it here

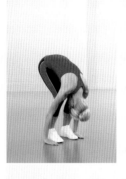

7 Dip-kick with twist With arms by your sides, bend both knees, then come up and kick one foot forward. Repeat for a total of 8 reps, then add a twist by turning your upper body and swinging the opposite arm to the kicking leg. Keep the arms shoulder-height. Keep your hips square. Repeat, alternating sides, for a total of 8 reps.

8 Roll-up Stand tall with feet hip-width apart, arms stretched above your head, shoulders relaxed, and neck and spine in line. Slowly lower your arms and take your chin towards your chest, then round your back and slowly bend down towards the floor. When you are as low as possible, your hands should be relaxed and as near to the floor as is comfortable. Take a deep breath into your lower back. Then, keeping your tummy pulled into your lower back, uncurl slowly, one vertebra at a time, until you have returned to a standing position.

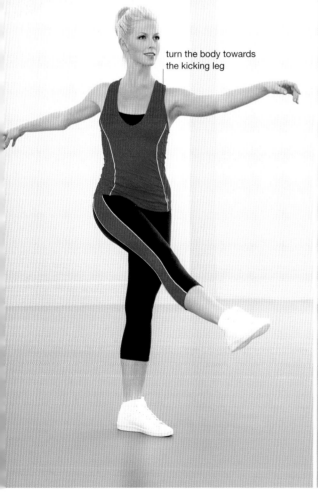

turn the body towards the kicking leg

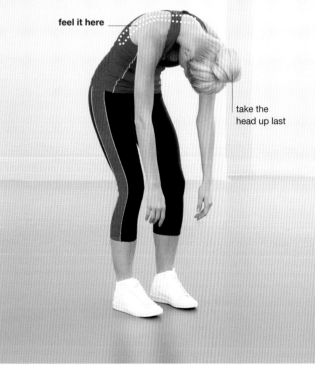

feel it here

take the head up last

>> **workout** march/jog

9 **March** Standing on one foot, raise the other knee to waist-height. At the same time, raise the opposite arm. March on the spot, raising opposite knees and arms. Repeat for a total of 16 reps.

10 **Jog** Curling the opposite arm to the lifted foot, jog on the spot, raising your heels towards your buttocks. Make sure your heels touch the ground every time you land. Repeat for a total of 16 reps.

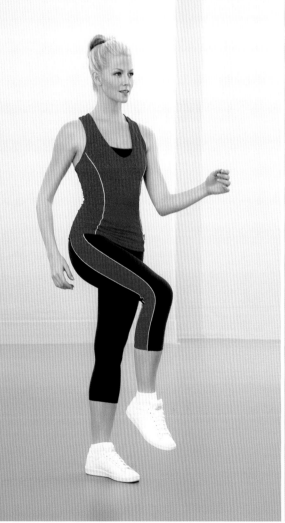

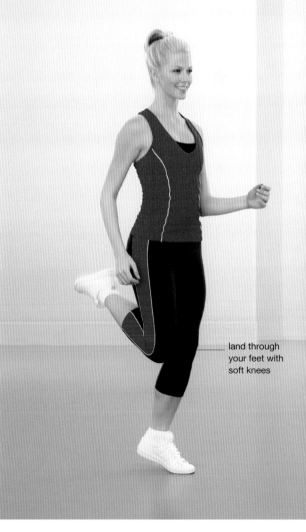

land through
your feet with
soft knees

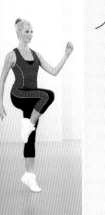

11 **Sprint start** Lift one knee towards your chest as you come up onto the toes of the other foot. As you do this, raise the arm opposite to your lifted knee to shoulder-height. The other arm is held slightly behind the body with the elbow soft. Replace the lifted leg to the floor, taking the foot slightly behind and with the knee bent, as you transfer your weight forward. Lift the toe of the opposite leg to flex the foot. Reverse the arms. Repeat for a total of 8 reps, then change sides and repeat for a total of 8 reps.

12 **Knees up** Jump from one leg to the other, lifting your knees high towards your chest. Pump with the opposite arms, so your arm is bent at the elbow and forward on the side of the supporting leg, and slightly bent and backward on the side of the raised knee. Make sure your heels touch the ground every time you land. Repeat for a total of 16 reps. Repeat Step 10.

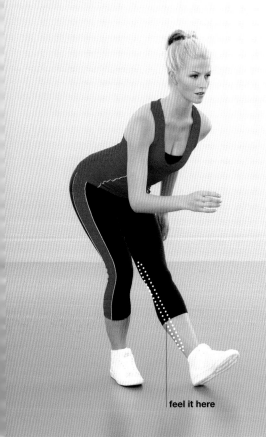

feel it here

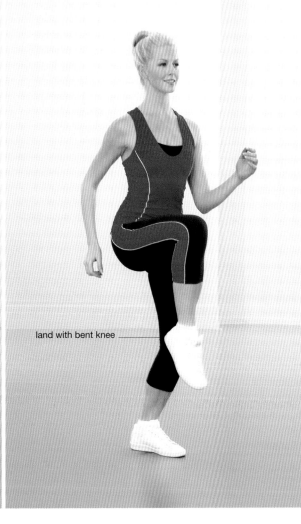

land with bent knee

13 **Ski run** Starting with both feet together, take a diagonal step forward and swing your arms across your body in the same direction. Bring the second foot to the first, then step to the other side and swing your arms the other way. Keep your knees bent and your body low to the ground. Take 4 steps forward, alternating from side to side in a skiing motion, then take 4 steps back in the same way for a total of 8 reps.

14 **Half jack** Starting with both feet together, hands by your sides, and elbows slightly bent, keep one foot planted and step to the side with the other. At the same time, raise both arms above your head. Lower your arms as you bring the foot at the side back to centre, then step to the other side to repeat. Repeat, alternating sides, for a total of 8 reps.

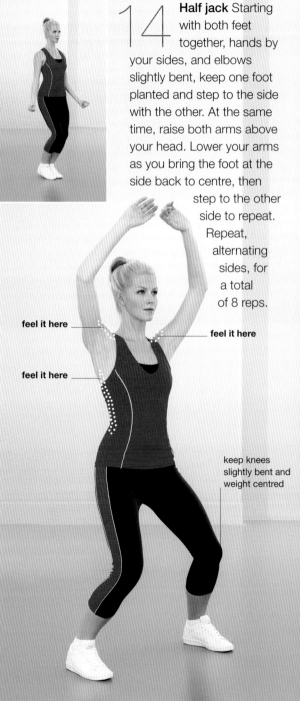

feel it here

feel it here

feel it here

keep knees slightly bent and weight centred

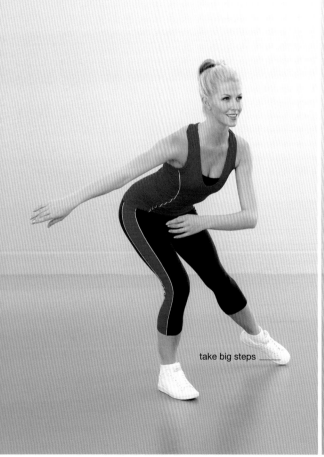

take big steps

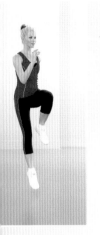

15 **Sprint-start jump**
Starting with both feet together, hop on one foot as you raise the other knee towards your chest. As you do this, raise the arm opposite to your lifted knee to shoulder-height. The other arm is held slightly behind the body with the elbow soft. Replace the lifted leg to the floor, taking the foot slightly behind and with the knee bent, as you transfer your weight forward. Lift the toe of the opposite leg to flex the foot. Reverse the arms. Repeat for a total of 8 reps, then change sides and repeat for a total of 8 reps. Repeat Step 10.

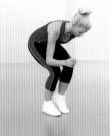

16 **Step pump**
Starting with both feet together, step forward, crouching over one leg with the heel of the other foot raised. Your arm on the side of the raised heel swings slightly behind your body. Your other arm is bent at the elbow. Lower the raised heel as you step back on that foot to an upright position and straighten the other leg. Reverse the arms. Repeat for a total of 8 reps, then change sides and repeat for a total of 8 reps.

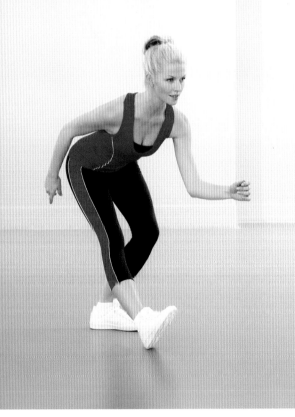

>> **workout** lunge/ski run with hop

17 **Lunge** Starting with both feet together, hands on hips, step forward on one foot into a lunge position. Come up, bringing your feet back together, then repeat on the other side. Make sure your hips are square and your knees are in line with your toes. Keep your back straight and your neck and spine in line. Repeat, alternating sides, for a total of 4 reps.

18 **Ski run with hop** Starting with both feet together, take a diagonal step forward, adding a little hop, and swinging your arms across your body in the same direction. Bring the second foot to the first, then step and hop to the other side, swinging your arms the other way. Keep your knees bent and your body low to the ground. Take 4 steps forward, alternating from side to side in a skiing motion, then take 4 steps back in the same way for a total of 8 reps.

Repeat Step 10, then Steps 9–12, then Step 10 again, then Steps 13–15, then Step 10 again, then Steps 16–18, and finally, Step 10 again.

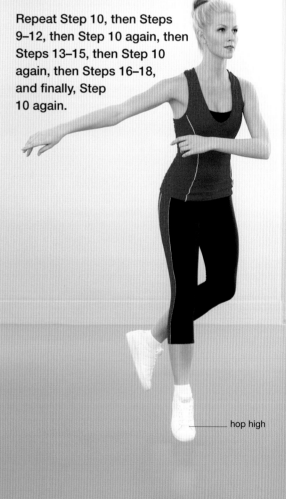

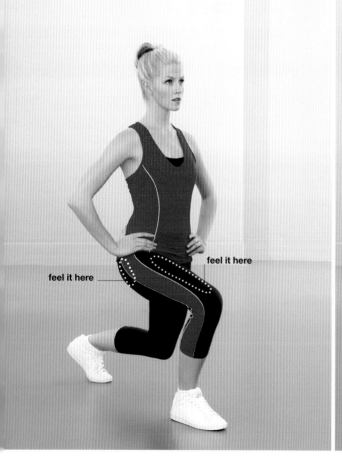

feel it here

feel it here

hop high

19 **March** Standing on one foot, raise the other knee to hip-height. At the same time, raise the opposite arm. March on the spot, raising opposite knees and arms. Repeat for a total of 24 reps.

20 **Three-in-one stretch 1** Keeping both toes pointing forward, take one leg behind you, and bend the front knee. Clasp your hands in front and raise your arms towards your ears as you lower your head. You should feel a stretch in your upper back, neck, and calf.

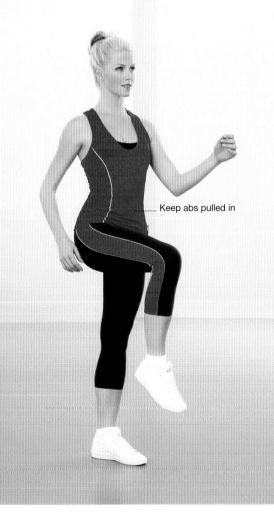

Keep abs pulled in

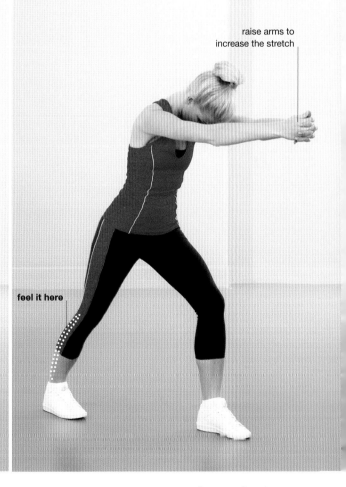

raise arms to increase the stretch

feel it here

>> **cool down** 3-in-1 stretch 2/quad stretch

21 **Three-in-one stretch 2** Take the other leg behind, toes pointing forward, and front knee bent. Clasp your hands behind your back. Open your chest as you raise your arms behind you. You should feel a stretch in your calf, chest, and arms.

22 **Quad stretch** Stand on one leg and hold the other foot with the hand on the same side. Bring the heel of the raised foot towards the buttock until you feel a stretch in the front of the bent-leg thigh. Change legs. If you cannot keep your balance, hold onto a support.

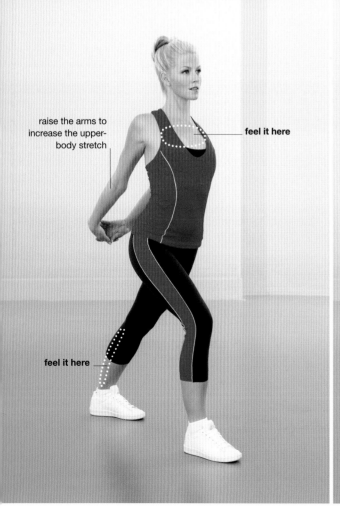

raise the arms to increase the upper-body stretch

feel it here

feel it here

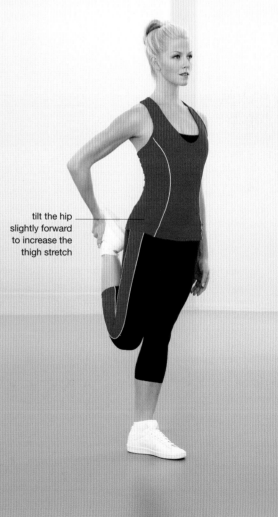

tilt the hip slightly forward to increase the thigh stretch

23 **Inner-thigh stretch** Take a step to one side and bend that knee, keeping the knee directly over the toes. Take your hands to the bent-leg thigh and lean forward, stretching the other leg out to the side. Make sure your neck and spine stay in line, and keep your back long and straight. You should feel a stretch in the inner thigh of the outstretched leg. Repeat on the other side.

24 **Roll-up** Stand tall with feet hip-width apart, arms stretched above your head, shoulders relaxed, and neck and spine in line. Slowly lower your arms and take your chin towards your chest, then round your back and slowly bend down towards the floor. When you are as low as possible, your hands should be relaxed and as near to the floor as is comfortable. Take a deep breath into your lower back. Then, keeping your tummy pulled into your lower back, uncurl slowly, one vertebra at a time, until you have returned to a standing position.

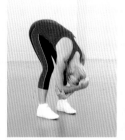

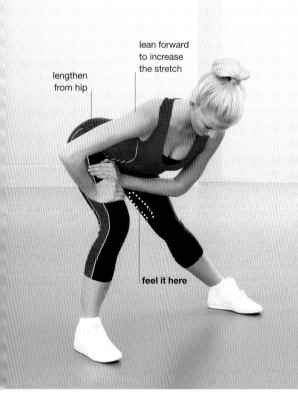

lengthen from hip

lean forward to increase the stretch

feel it here

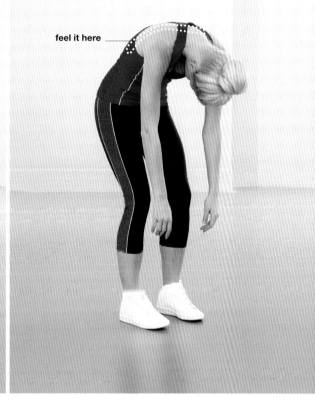

feel it here

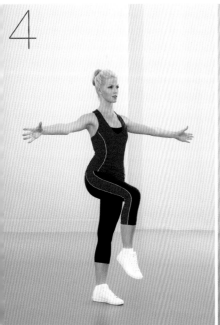

▲ **Warm up** March and flick,
page 71

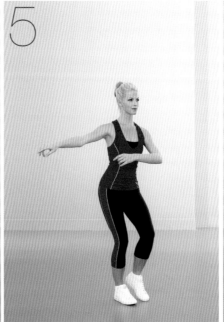

▲ **Warm up** Side step,
page 72

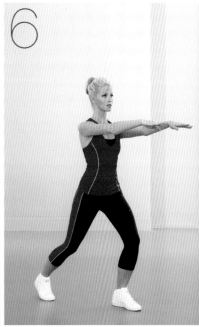

▲ **Warm up** Back step,
page 72

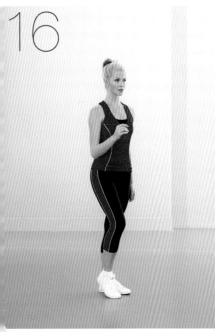

▲ **Workout** Step pump,
page 77

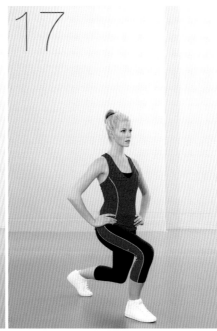

▲ **Workout** Lunge,
page 78

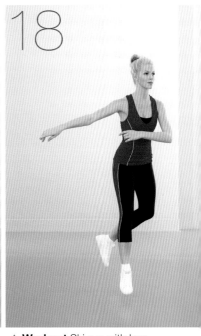

▲ **Workout** Ski-run with hop,
page 78

running workout at a glance

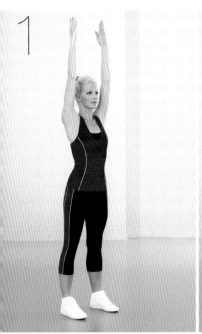

1

▲ **Warm up** Deep breaths,
page 70

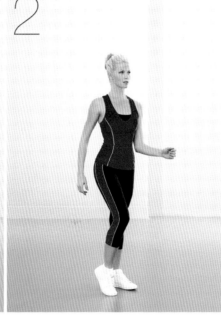

2

▲ **Warm up** Half-toe pump,
page 70

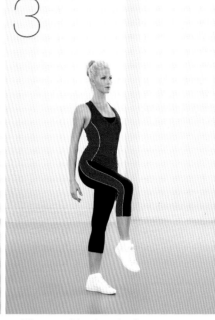

3

▲ **Warm up** March and roll,
page 71

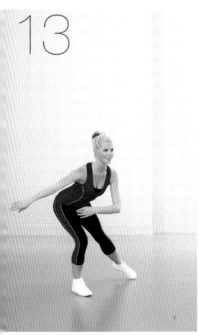

13

▲ **Workout** Ski-run,
page 76

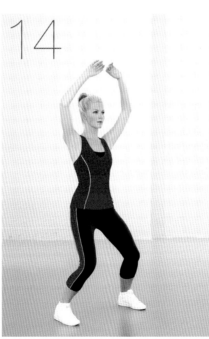

14

▲ **Workout** Half jack,
page 76

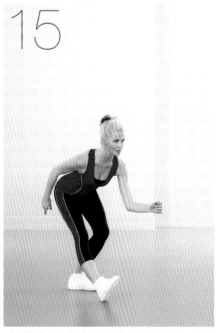

15

▲ **Workout** Sprint-start jump,
page 77

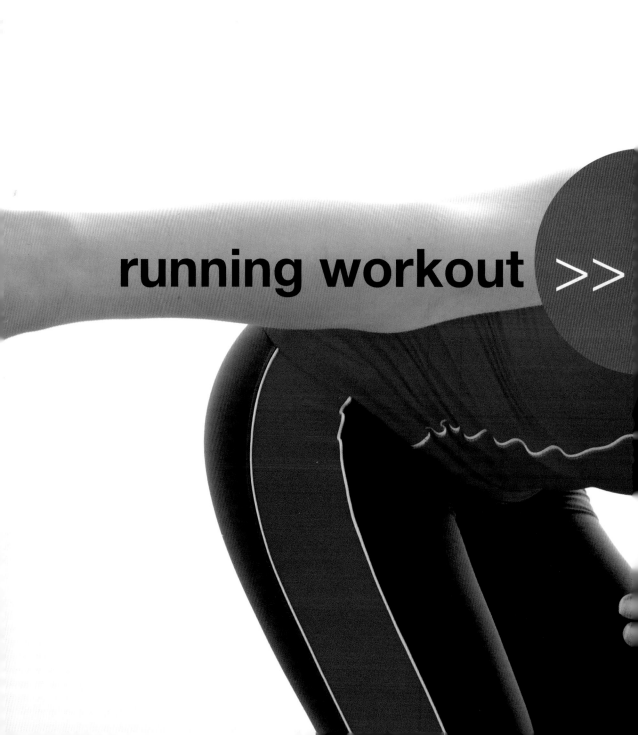

running workout >>

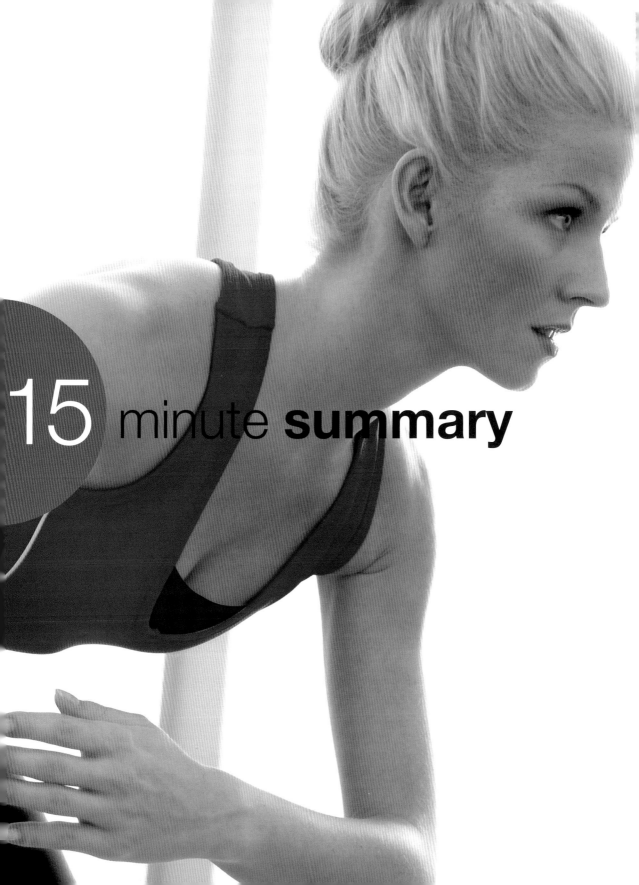

15 minute **summary**

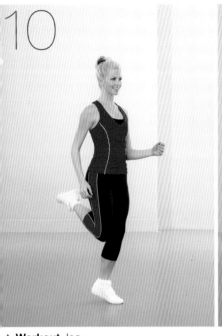

10

▲ **Workout** Jog,
page 74

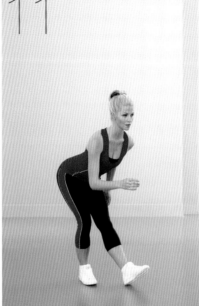

11

▲ **Workout** Sprint start,
page 75

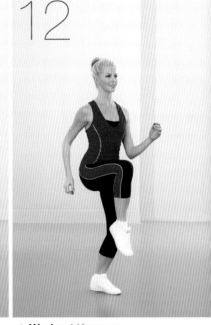

12

▲ **Workout** Knees up,
page 75

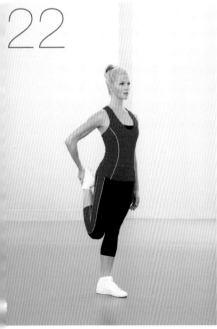

22

▲ **Cool down** Quad stretch,
page 80

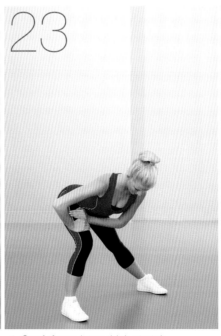

23

▲ **Cool down** Inner-thigh stretch,
page 81

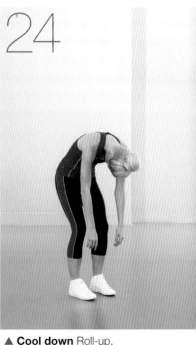

24

▲ **Cool down** Roll-up,
page 81

7

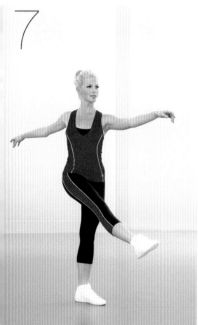

▲ **Warm up** Dip-kick with twist, page 73

8

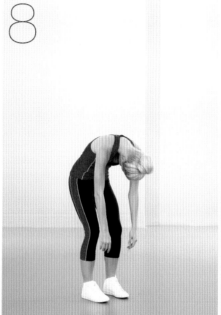

▲ **Warm up** Roll-up, page 73

9

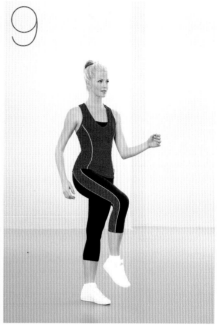

▲ **Workout** March, page 74

19

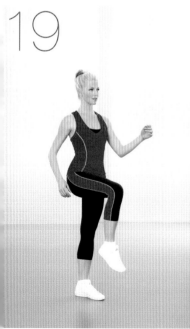

▲ **Cool down** March, page 79

20

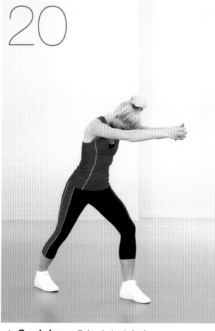

▲ **Cool down** 3-in-1stretch 1, page 79

21

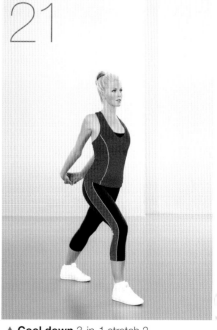

▲ **Cool down** 3-in-1 stretch 2, page 80

>> **running workout** FAQs

Running is a high-intensity form of exercise, and this sequence aims to match that. When working this hard and doing high-impact steps like jogging, take care to work correctly. You need very little space to perform this workout successfully, but if you have more, use it.

>> Does this sequence give me as much of a workout as if I were running outside?

In this sequence you are working very differently from outdoor running, mainly because you are on the spot most of the time and not having to cover any ground. Fifteen minutes of this workout will probably burn slightly fewer calories than running outside or on a treadmill, but it has the added bonus of giving you much more sculpting and toning of your muscles.

>> Can I do full Jacks instead of the Half jacks described in the sequence?

By all means. Full Jacks – also known as Star jumps and Jumping jacks – in which you jump instead of step, will make this step high-impact and will keep you working harder. If you are going for this option, make sure you land softly through your legs, with your knees over your toes. Your arms should follow the same pattern of movement as in the Half jacks.

>> I feel a burning sensation in the back of my lower leg when I do this Running sequence. Why is that and what can I do to make it go away?

This is your calf muscle and it is probably feeling like this because it is absorbing too much impact when you land. Make sure when you are jogging, jumping, or doing any other high-impact movement, that you land with your knees soft, and that your heels come down lightly when you land.

>> What is the aim of the March?

This may seem like a very simple step and not very taxing, so to make sure you are getting the most from it, take your knees up and really use your arms – lifting your knees to hip-height or above and swinging your arms at least as high as your shoulders. Bearing in mind that you have to return your foot to the floor before the other leg comes up, you should be making pretty big movements to get up and back in time. Only you will know if you are marching as intensively as you can. The intensity of this step is so easily modified that I have also used it as a component for my Warm Up and Cool Down sections. Remember and recognize which section you are marching in!

>> I can't seem to add the hop to the Ski runs with hop, and still keep in time. What can I do to get it right?

The "hop" is part of the step forward, so you need to step forward and push off the foot in one movement as opposed to stepping, landing, and then trying to hop after that. The more of a bend you can get in your knee as you step forward, the more you will be able to use that to push off, and in that way get bigger and higher hops.

>> I find the Lunges very uncomfortable and can't do them all as my legs hurt. Does that matter?

Form is even more important than usual on this exercise, which is one of the reasons it is performed more slowly than the others. Make sure you keep lifting from your waist and watch your posture. Your weight should be centred evenly between your legs so you are not giving them a dead weight to carry. Make sure you try to "power" from your bottom as opposed to your thighs. If all else fails, cut the number of reps until you've got used to the move.

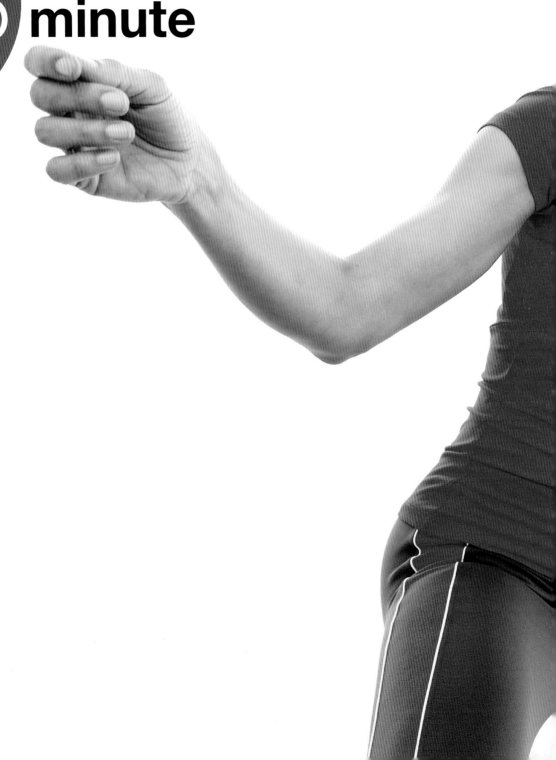

15 minute

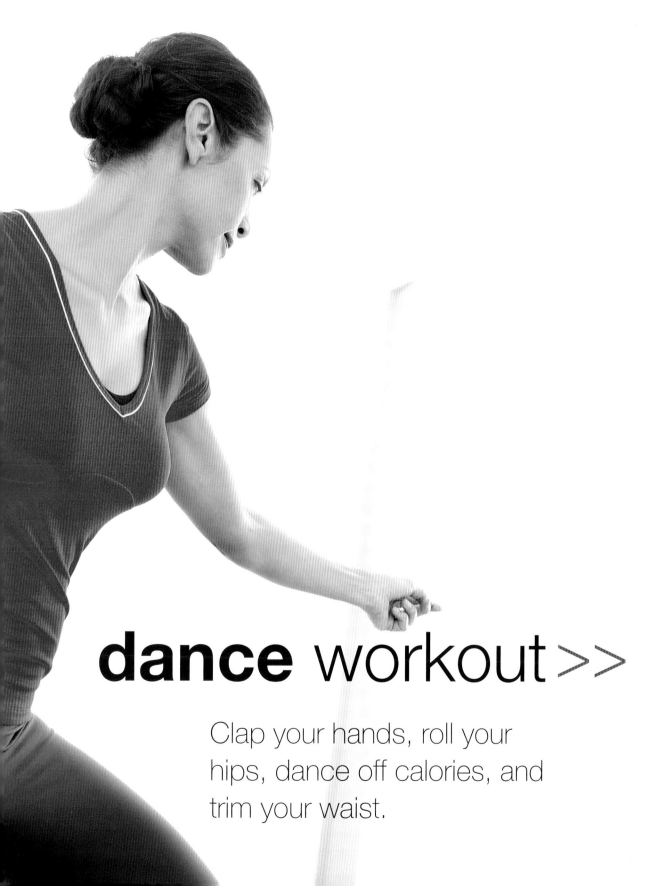

dance workout >>

Clap your hands, roll your hips, dance off calories, and trim your waist.

>> **dance** workout

I met someone a long time ago who had developed his own workout. Every day he went to his local park, put on his headphones and danced freestyle for an hour to his favourite music. That's what dancing should be all about, so have fun. Dance this sequence like no one is watching!

There are many different styles of dance and dance training – and they are all constantly changing and evolving – so I'm not even going to attempt to list them or compare the benefits of one with another. Suffice it to say that for this particular sequence, I've borrowed moves from two of my favourite dance styles – disco and reggae. These moves are designed not only for the enjoyment they offer, but also for their good aerobic workout. And you'll certainly appreciate their waist-trimming effect and how they burn the calories.

The best way to intensify this workout and burn extra calories is to let yourself go and really dance your heart out. You'll be surprised how much fun you have and how quickly you feel you've had a worthwhile workout.

Another way is to maintain your posture and form throughout. One thing you will notice about accomplished and professional dancers, regardless of what style of dance they do, is their beautiful posture. Not only does any movement look better when executed with good form and great posture, but it also has a much more beneficial effect on the body in terms of toning and working core muscles.

In fact, a professional dancer's beautiful posture comes from years of core training – strengthening the lower and upper back, and working all the abdominal muscles, including all the deep muscles we can't see. Try to emulate the professionals and you won't fail to burn extra calories. Keep up the effort in your everyday life, and you'll soon notice the difference.

>> **tips for** my dance workout

- **As with all training and exercise,** you get back what you put in, so even though this workout may appear to be pretty relaxed, do keep working, stay focused, and really twist your waist.

- **Dancing with company** can boost your fun, so try this dance workout with a friend or partner.

- **Forget you are** even doing any "exercise". Dancing is such an informal way of working your body – especially this relaxed style – so it shouldn't be a chore!

This workout also gives you plenty of opportunity for adding your own special flavour. As soon as you feel you've got the hang of the basic steps, go ahead and add a little hop, or a "shake", or a hand clap. Make it your own. Keep moving. Have a good time. Persuade a friend or partner to get involved, too, and if you've small children, perhaps you can share the moves with them. Watching them doing their own version of the steps can be priceless!

A dance workout can help you develop and tone your core muscles. It strengthens your upper and lower back, and works wonders for your abdominal muscles, too.

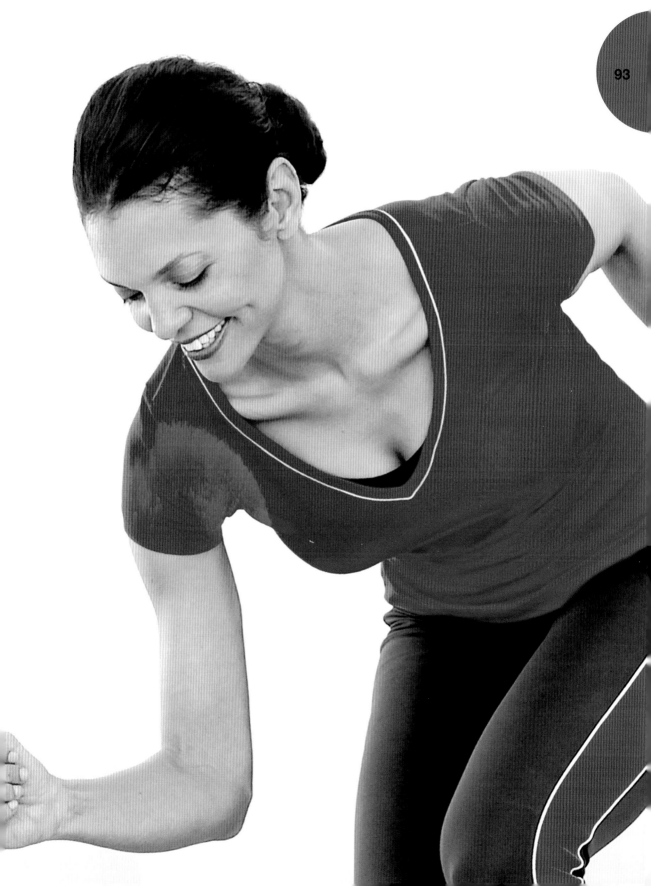

>> **warm up** deep breaths/half-toe pump

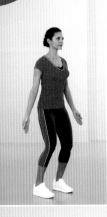

1 **Deep breaths** Stand tall with feet hip-width apart, knees soft, and arms by your sides. Relax your neck and shoulders, and make sure your tummy is pulled in. Take a deep breath in as you bend the knees and raise your arms above your head. Exhale as you lower them with a smooth circular movement. Make sure your back stays straight. Repeat for a total of 4 reps.

2 **Half-toe pump** Alternate your weight from one foot to the other, rising up onto the ball of your foot. As you alternate feet, curl the opposite arm to your shoulder. Keep your hands in a loose fist and make sure you push your heel right down to the floor as you work your calf muscle. Repeat for a total of 16 reps (1 rep = both sides/directions).

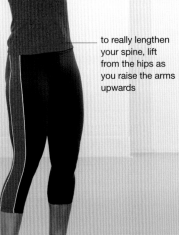

to really lengthen your spine, lift from the hips as you raise the arms upwards

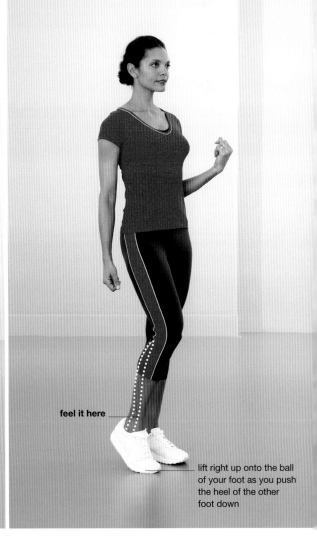

feel it here

lift right up onto the ball of your foot as you push the heel of the other foot down

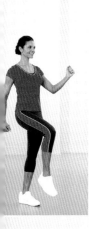

3 **March and roll** Standing on one foot, raise the other knee to waist-height. At the same time, raise the opposite arm. March on the spot, raising opposite knees and arms. Repeat for a total of 8 reps. Then, with your arms by your sides, raise your shoulders towards your ears and roll them in a circular motion, backwards, then forwards. Repeat for a total of 4 reps.

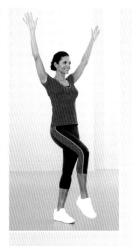

4 **March and flick** Continue marching and, as you do so, stretch your arms sideways to meet above your head, opening and closing your hands at intervals with a "flicking" motion, to warm your fingers and wrists. Continue "flicking" your hands as you lower your arms. Repeat for a total of 4 reps.

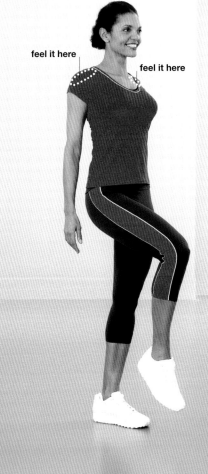

feel it here

feel it here

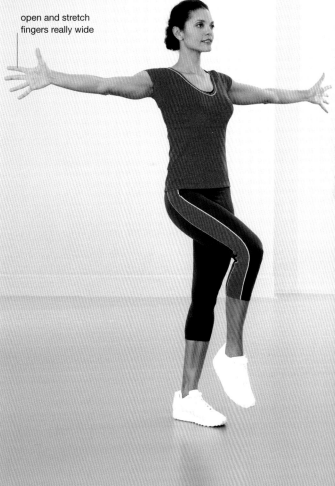

open and stretch fingers really wide

>> **warm up** side step/back step

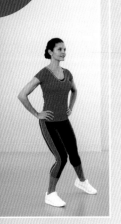

5 **Side step** With hands on hips, take a step to one side, then bring your feet together. Repeat to the other side. Repeat for a total of 4 reps, then swing your arms in the same direction as you are stepping. Your arms should be relaxed and raised no higher than shoulder-height. Repeat for a total of 8 reps.

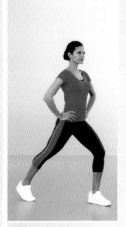

6 **Back step** With hands on hips, touch one foot on the floor behind you. Return to centre. Repeat with the opposite foot. Keep your weight centred as you alternate legs. Repeat for a total of 4 reps, then add an arm push in time with your leg movements by pushing both arms forward and back just below shoulder-height. Repeat for a total of 8 reps.

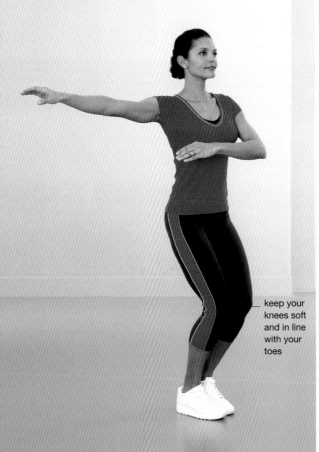

keep your knees soft and in line with your toes

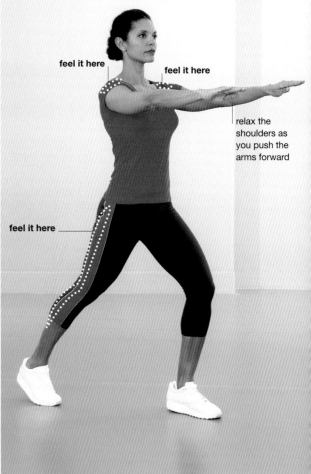

feel it here

feel it here

relax the shoulders as you push the arms forward

feel it here

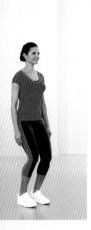

7 **Dip-kick with twist** With arms by your sides, bend both knees, then come up and kick one foot forward. Repeat for a total of 8 reps, then add a twist by turning your upper body and swinging the opposite arm to the kicking leg. Keep the arms shoulder-height. Keep your hips square. Repeat, alternating sides, for a total of 8 reps.

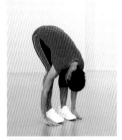

8 **Roll-up** Stand tall with feet hip-width apart, arms stretched above your head, shoulders relaxed, and neck and spine in line. Slowly lower your arms and take your chin towards your chest, then round your back and slowly bend down towards the floor. When you are as low as possible, your hands should be relaxed and as near to the floor as is comfortable. Take a deep breath into your lower back. Then, keeping your tummy pulled into your lower back, uncurl slowly, one vertebra at a time, until you have returned to a standing position.

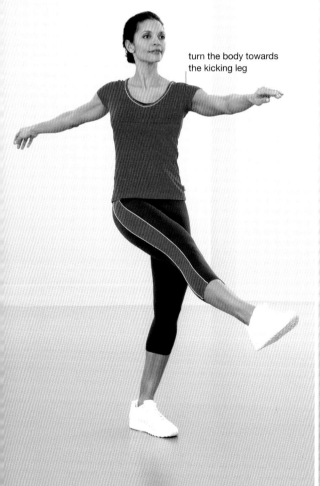

turn the body towards the kicking leg

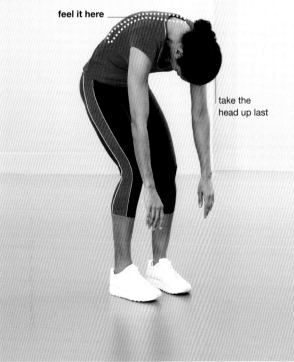

feel it here

take the head up last

>> **workout** the swivel/ step dig

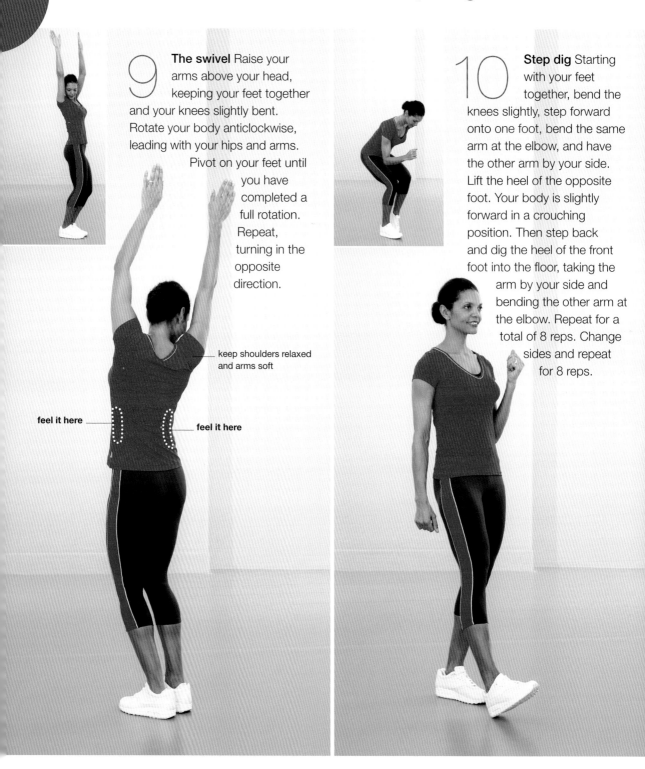

9 **The swivel** Raise your arms above your head, keeping your feet together and your knees slightly bent. Rotate your body anticlockwise, leading with your hips and arms. Pivot on your feet until you have completed a full rotation. Repeat, turning in the opposite direction.

keep shoulders relaxed and arms soft

feel it here

feel it here

10 **Step dig** Starting with your feet together, bend the knees slightly, step forward onto one foot, bend the same arm at the elbow, and have the other arm by your side. Lift the heel of the opposite foot. Your body is slightly forward in a crouching position. Then step back and dig the heel of the front foot into the floor, taking the arm by your side and bending the other arm at the elbow. Repeat for a total of 8 reps. Change sides and repeat for 8 reps.

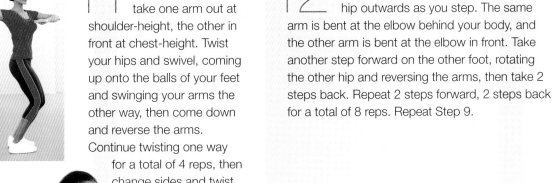

11 **Twist and shift** With the feet together, take one arm out at shoulder-height, the other in front at chest-height. Twist your hips and swivel, coming up onto the balls of your feet and swinging your arms the other way, then come down and reverse the arms. Continue twisting one way for a total of 4 reps, then change sides and twist the other way for a total of 4 reps. Repeat.

12 **Step roll** Starting with the feet together, step forward onto one toe, rotating your hip outwards as you step. The same arm is bent at the elbow behind your body, and the other arm is bent at the elbow in front. Take another step forward on the other foot, rotating the other hip and reversing the arms, then take 2 steps back. Repeat 2 steps forward, 2 steps back for a total of 8 reps. Repeat Step 9.

feel it here ———

——— **feel it here**

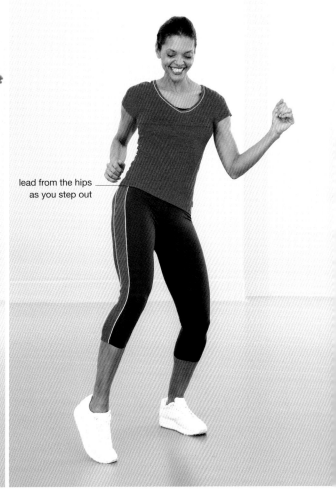

lead from the hips ———
as you step out

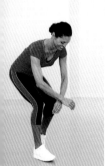

13 **Step dig and clap** Step forward as you crouch over the front leg, both knees bent, and touching the toes of the back foot to the floor. Cross your arms in front of your knees. Step back onto the other leg, digging the front heel into the floor and at the same time raising your hands above your head and clapping. Step backwards and forwards for a total of 8 reps, then step forward onto the other foot and repeat.

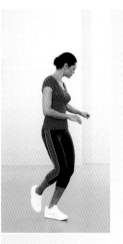

14 **The rock** Step one leg forward, allowing the other leg to come up onto its toes and bend at the knee. With your elbows bent, let your hands follow the forward step at hip-height. Return that foot to centre and swing your arms the other way. Count "1, 2, 3". Repeat with the other leg. Repeat for a total of 6 reps.

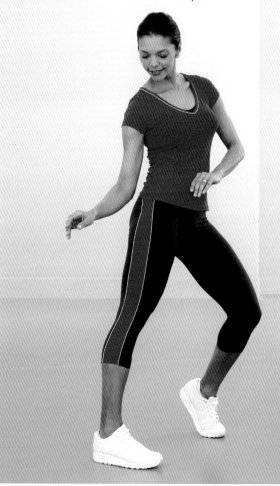

15 **Step hop** Hop onto one leg, raising the opposite knee. Swing the opposite arm forward to shoulder-height and the other arm back. Hop onto the other leg, swinging the arms the other way. Your upper body should follow the motion of the arms as you alternate from side to side. Repeat for a total of 8 reps. Repeat Step 9.

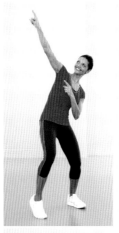

16 **Side-step point** Take a step to one side, keeping the other heel raised as you point skywards in the direction of the step. Swing the other arm across your body. Lower your arms to point to the floor as you bring your feet together. Repeat to the same side, then repeat by taking 2 steps to the other side. Repeat, alternating sides, for a total of 8 reps.

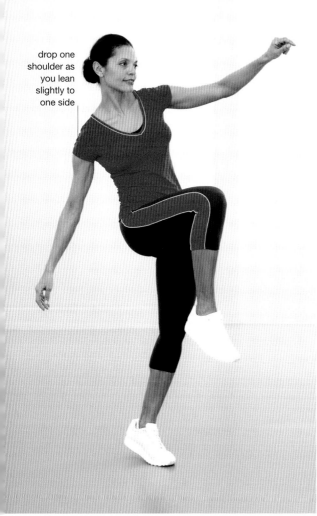

drop one shoulder as you lean slightly to one side

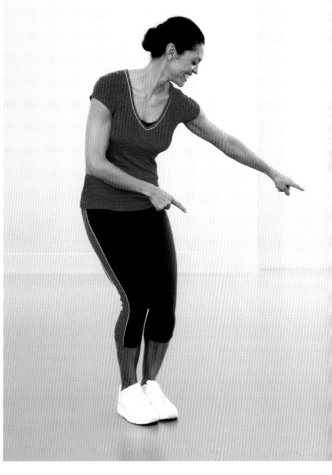

>> **workout** heel-dig pump/side-dig swing

17 **Heel-dig pump** Starting with feet together, dig one heel forward and raise the toes. Curl the opposite arm to shoulder-height. Repeat, alternating sides, for a total of 16 reps.

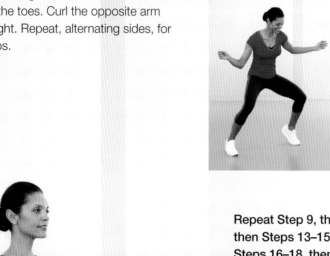

18 **Side-dig swing** Starting with feet together, step to one side, opening both arms out to the sides at chest-height. Return that foot to centre, bending your arms and crossing them in front of your body at waist-height, then repeat to the other side. Repeat, alternating sides, for a total of 8 reps.

Repeat Step 9, then Steps 10-12, then Step 9, then Steps 13–15, then Step 9, then Steps 16–18, then Step 9, then Steps 10-12 again, and finally, Step 9 again.

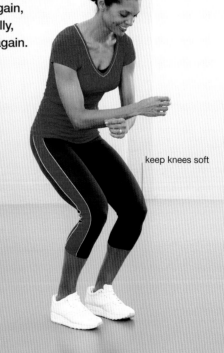

keep knees soft

19 **March** Standing on one foot, raise the other knee to hip-height. At the same time, raise the opposite arm. March on the spot, raising opposite knees and arms. Repeat for a total of 24 reps.

20 **Three-in-one stretch 1** Keeping both toes pointing forward, take one leg behind you, and bend the front knee. Clasp your hands in front and raise your arms towards your ears as you lower your head. You should feel a stretch in your upper back, neck, and calf.

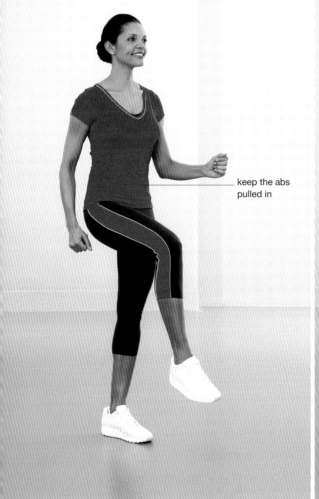

keep the abs pulled in

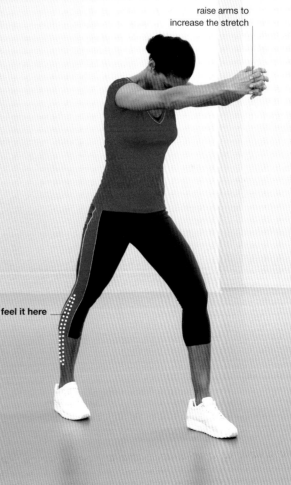

raise arms to increase the stretch

feel it here

21 **Three-in-one stretch 2** Take the other leg behind, toes pointing forward, and front knee bent. Clasp your hands behind your back. Open your chest as you raise your arms behind you. You should feel a stretch in your calf, chest, and arms.

22 **Quad stretch** Stand on one leg and hold the other foot with the hand on the same side. Bring the heel of the raised foot towards the buttock until you feel a stretch in the front of the bent-leg thigh. Change legs. If you cannot keep your balance, hold onto a support.

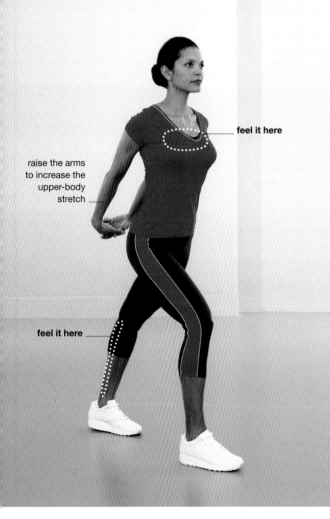

feel it here

raise the arms
to increase the
upper-body
stretch

feel it here

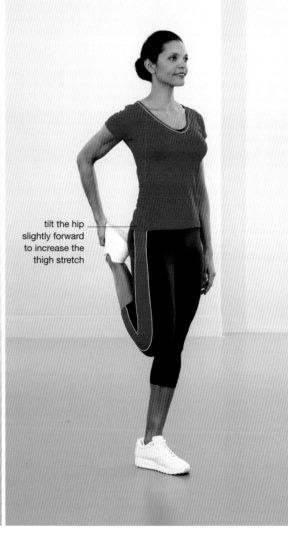

tilt the hip
slightly forward
to increase the
thigh stretch

23 **Inner-thigh stretch** Take a step to one side and bend that knee, keeping the knee directly over the toes. Take your hands to the bent-leg thigh and lean forward, stretching the other leg out to the side. Make sure your neck and spine stay in line, and keep your back long and straight. You should feel a stretch in the inner thigh of the outstretched leg. Repeat on the other side.

24 **Roll-up** Stand tall with feet hip-width apart, arms stretched above your head, shoulders relaxed, and neck and spine in line. Slowly lower your arms and take your chin towards your chest, then round your back and slowly bend down towards the floor. When you are as low as possible, your hands should be relaxed and as near to the floor as is comfortable. Take a deep breath into your lower back. Then, keeping your tummy pulled into your lower back, uncurl slowly, one vertebra at a time, until you have returned to a standing position.

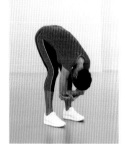

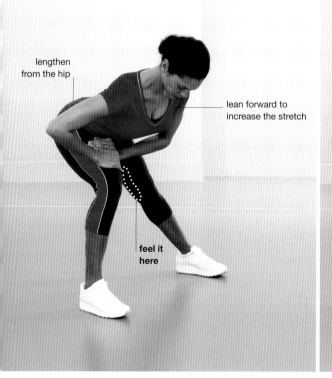

lengthen from the hip

lean forward to increase the stretch

feel it here

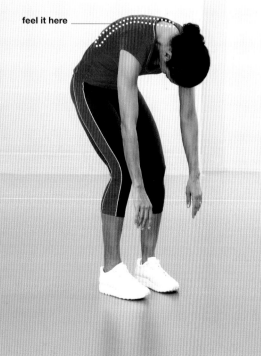

feel it here

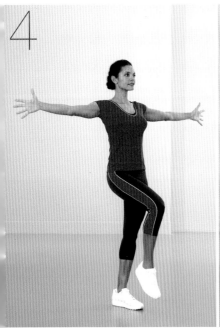

▲ **Warm up** March and flick,
page 95

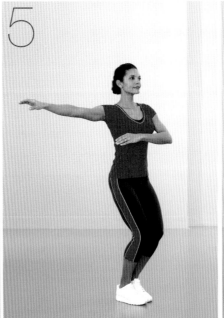

▲ **Warm up** Side step,
page 96

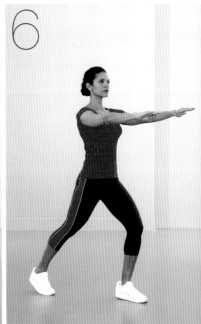

▲ **Warm up** Back step,
page 96

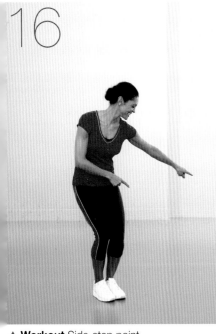

▲ **Workout** Side-step point,
page 101

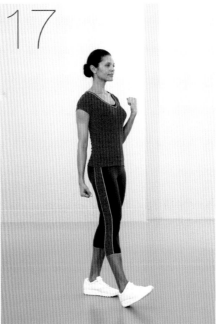

▲ **Workout** Heel-dig pump,
page 102

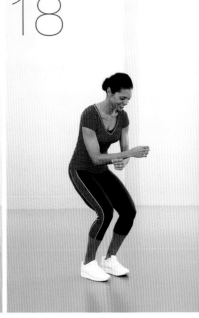

▲ **Workout** Side-dig swing,
page 102

dance workout at a glance

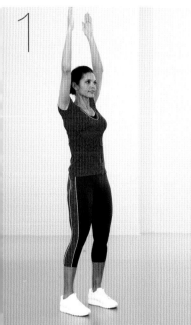

▲ **Warm up** Deep breaths,
page 94

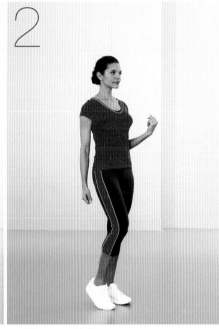

▲ **Warm up** Half-toe pump,
page 94

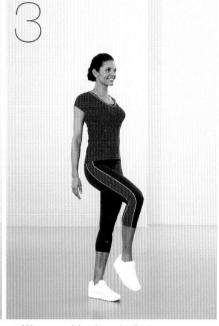

▲ **Warm up** March and roll,
page 95

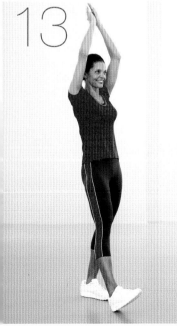

▲ **Workout** Step dig and clap,
page 100

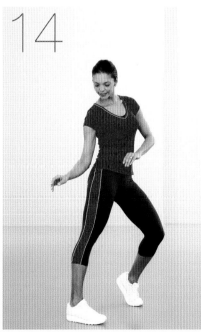

▲ **Workout** The rock,
page 100

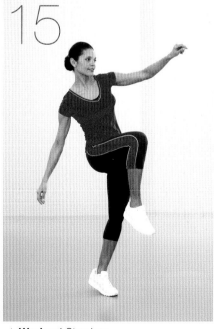

▲ **Workout** Step hop,
page 101

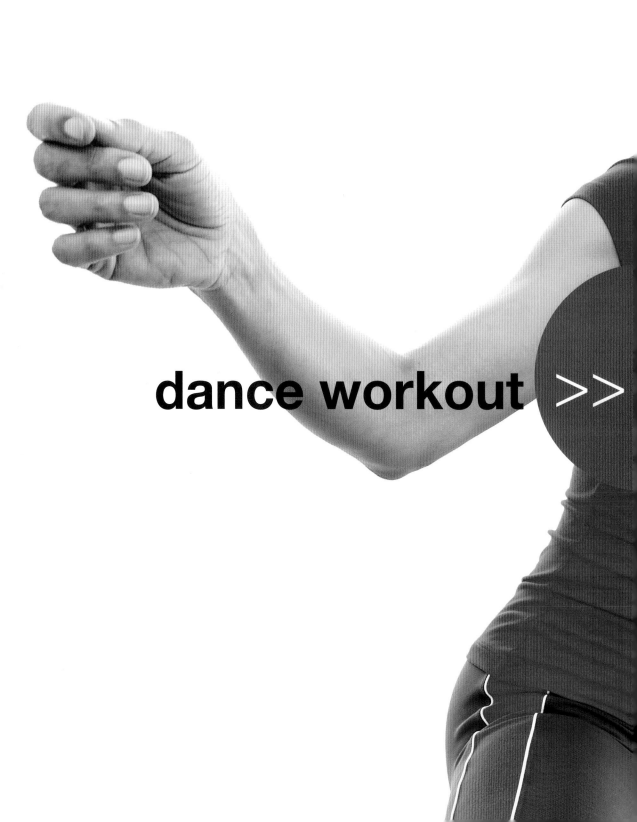

dance workout >>

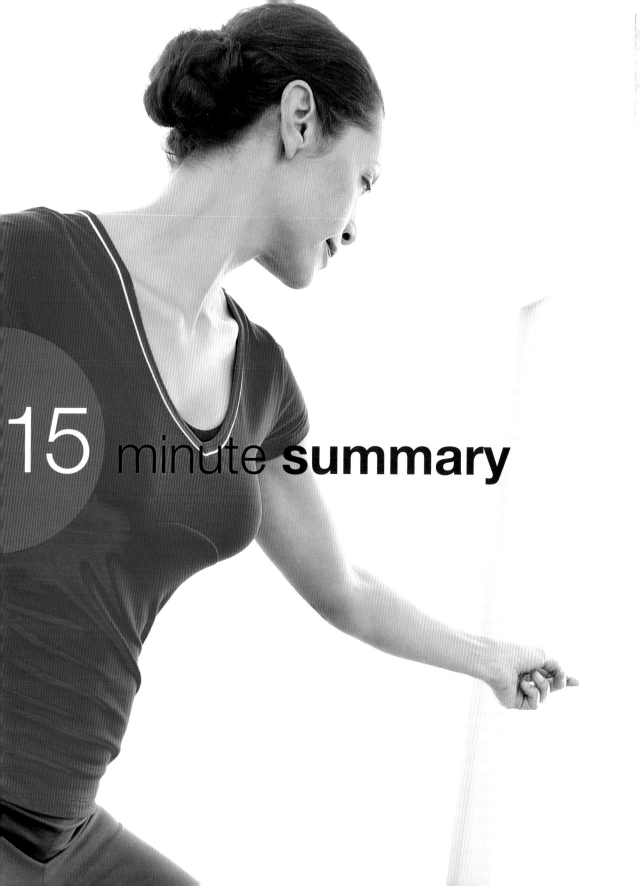

15 minute **summary**

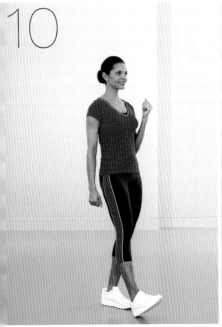

▲ **Workout** Step dig,
page 98

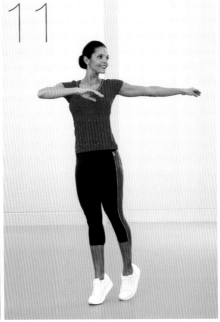

▲ **Workout** Twist and shift,
page 99

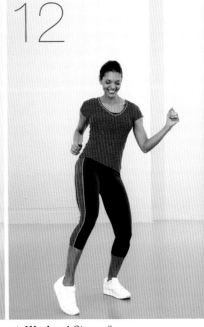

▲ **Workout** Step roll,
page 99

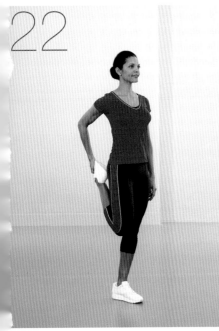

▲ **Cool down** Quad stretch,
page 104

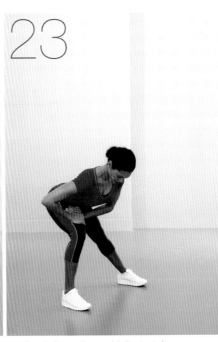

▲ **Cool down** Inner-thigh stretch,
page 105

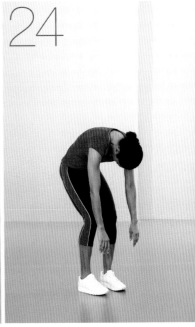

▲ **Cool down** Roll-up,
page 105

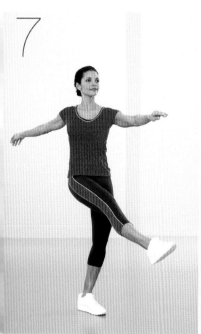

▲ **Warm up** Dip-kick with twist, page 97

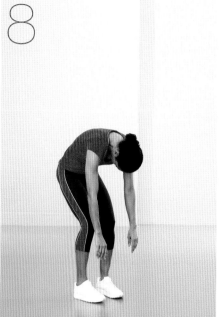

▲ **Warm up** Roll-up, page 97

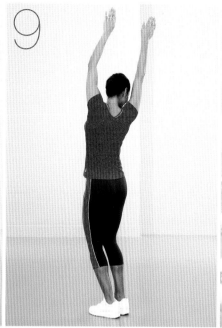

▲ **Workout** The swivel, page 98

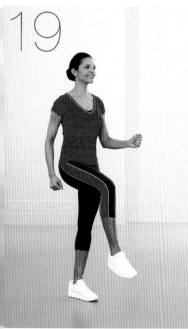

▲ **Cool down** March, page 103

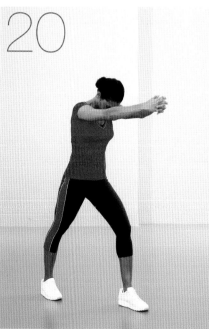

▲ **Cool down** 3-in-1 stretch 1, page 103

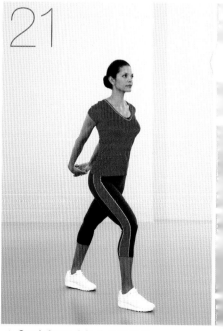

▲ **Cool down** 3-in-1 stretch 2, page 104

>> dance workout FAQs

Dancing is something we all do at some point, whether we're good at it or not. For this sequence I've selected steps which aren't difficult to master if you're a beginner, but they're also versatile and give you scope to add little touches of your own if you're more advanced.

>> Is there any area of the body in particular I am working in the Dance Workout?

Yes, your waist! Many of the moves in this sequence are designed to work that area, particularly The swivel. To reap maximum benefits, make sure your tummy is pulled in tight and you exaggerate the twist as you turn around.

>> What style of dance is this workout?

In short – a mix of a few. My training techniques draw on many different influences and this variety is reflected in the Dance Workout. Moves like The rock, and Step roll are classic "disco" steps. More traditional, with roots in "jazz dance", are steps like Side-step point, Step dig and Step dig and clap. Moves like The swivel and Step hop have more of an "urban" flavour.

>> I can't get the timing right when I'm doing The rock. Can you offer me some tips?

This can be a tricky one. It's an unusual step because you have to count it in threes, like a waltz, whereas you usually count most dance steps in even numbers – usually fours or eights. To get your timing right here, count: one, two, three, one, two, three ... as you move forwards and back.

>> I can't get the arm and leg coordination right when I do the Step dig. What am I doing wrong?

First of all try not to think about it so much, just as you don't think about your coordination when you are walking. Try the move without the arms first, and then let them follow naturally when you have learned the footwork. Remember, your focus is burning calories, so the more limbs you move at the same time the better, even if they are not yet following the exact plan!

>> I don't seem to travel at all when I'm doing The twist. Why is that?

This movement will not go very far on carpet! If you are on a smooth surface and are wearing appropriate footwear, you may be able to "swivel" your feet so you really do move from left to right. If you feel as if you are practically staying on the spot, do not be concerned. As long as you are focusing on twisting your waist and feeling that area working, you will be making progress.

>> Why do I get tired in my shoulders and arms when I am doing The swivel?

This is because you are not using correct form and so you are getting other muscle groups involved. Make sure you focus on your waist, and completely relax your shoulders before you lift up your arms. The arms do not have to be totally straight or in line with your head. Keep them soft and relaxed so you can concentrate on working your waist and enjoying your dancing.

>> Does the Dance Workout burn as many calories as the other exercise styles?

The Boxing and Running Workouts are more intense but, as with all exercise, what you put in determines what you get out. Maintain good form and posture, and take the movements to their maximum. Exaggerate the hops and swings. Make forward and back steps as big and wide as you can. The more enthusiastic you are, the more calories you will be able to burn!

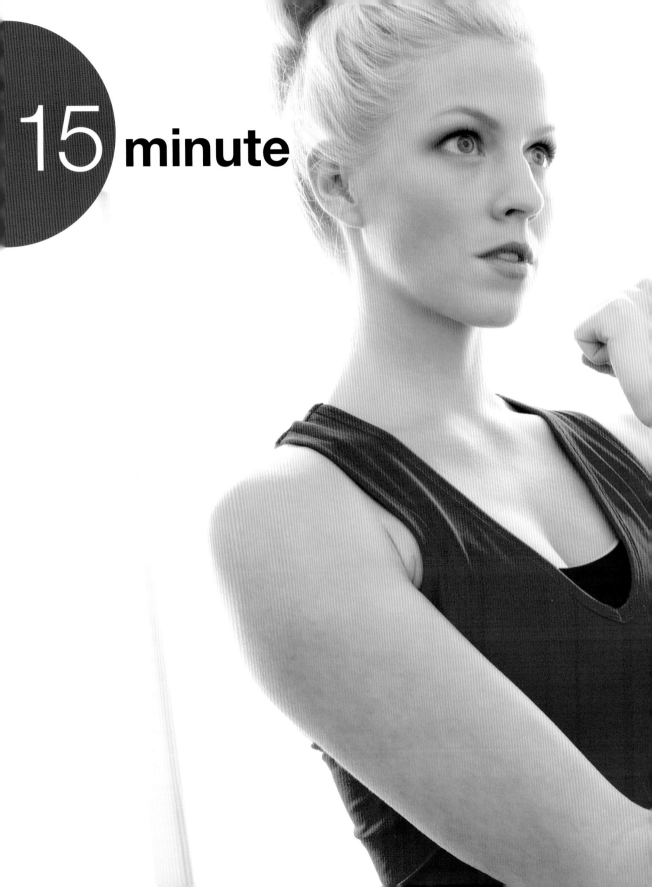

15 minute

moving on >>

The hardest step is the first, which you've taken. Now it's time to leave your comfort zone and move on to the next level.

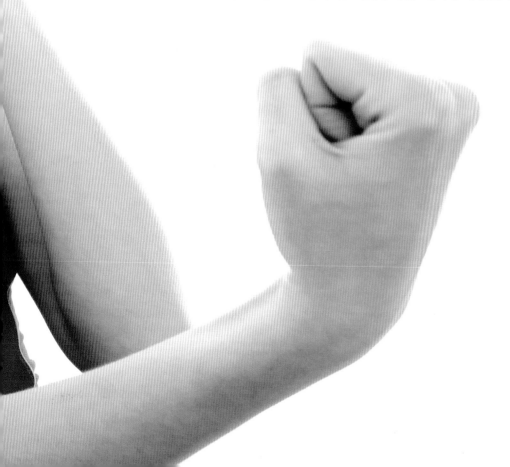

>> **boosting** the burn

You're exercising hard and avoiding foods with high sugar and fat contents, but somehow you're not losing the weight you want. The problem could be your metabolism. There are aspects of your metabolism that you can influence, so now is the time to work on those.

Metabolism refers to the chemical processes that go on in every cell of our body, enabling us to live and function. Controlled by our hormones and nervous system, metabolism keeps everything working as it should.

None of those chemical processes can take place without energy, and your body gets that, in the form of calories, from the food you eat.

Your Basal Metabolic Rate (BMR; see pp10–11) is the number of calories your body needs to sustain itself and to function – even when you're sleeping. You also need calories for all your physical activity, whether that's brushing your teeth or training for the Olympics. The bottom line is, if you want to lose weight, you must burn more calories than you take in (eat).

Burning more, burning less

Some of the factors that govern your BMR, such as your sex and age, are out of your control. If you're a man, your body needs more calories a day than if you are a woman. As you get older, your metabolism naturally slows down and uses fewer calories.

If you want to lose weight, you should target those factors you can control. One is your level of physical activity – more exercise burns more calories. The other is your lean-muscle-to-fat ratio. As it turns out, the two are linked. The more you exercise – particularly if you exercise in specific ways (see p119) – the more lean muscle you'll build, and having a high lean-muscle-to-fat ratio means you'll burn more calories (see p11). So it's a win-win situation.

>> **boost the burn** unusual facts

- **Too hot? Too cold?** If the ambient temperature is very low or very high, the body has to work harder to maintain its normal body temperature. Naturally enough, this increases your BMR.

- **Stand up for fitness.** Standing uses more energy than sitting, so next time you're standing on the bus, think of it as a mini-workout and enjoy it.

- **Time your eating.** Your metabolism is higher straight after exercise, so if you eat immediately after working out, you will burn more of those calories.

- **Fidgeting pays off.** An American study found that fidgeting produces "non exercise activity thermogenesis". In other words, it burns calories. People in the study with more body fat burned 350 calories less per day than those who were leaner. The leaner people fidgeted more and were generally more active.

- **The male advantage.** Men generally have faster metabolisms than women because they tend to be larger and have less body fat.

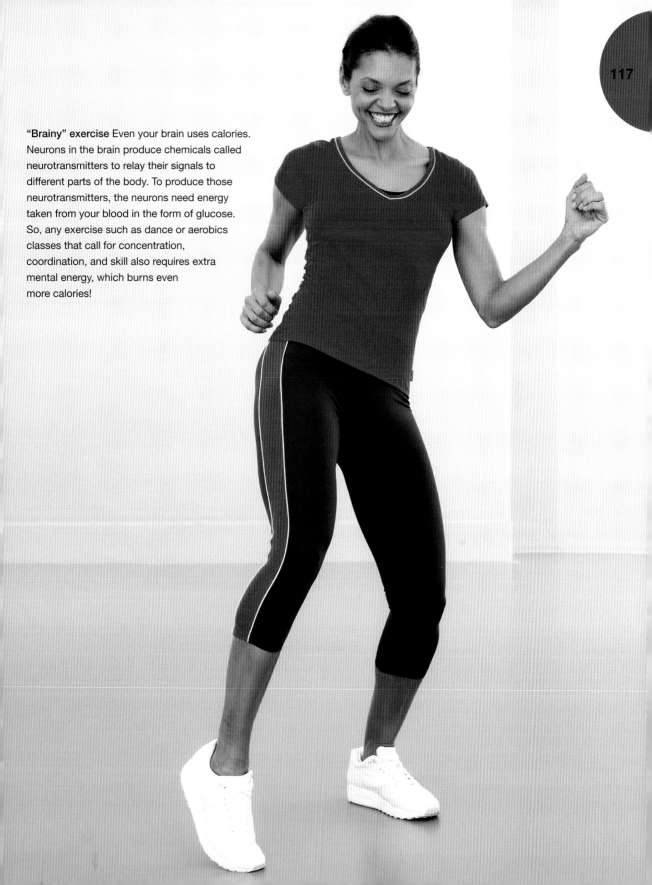

"Brainy" exercise Even your brain uses calories. Neurons in the brain produce chemicals called neurotransmitters to relay their signals to different parts of the body. To produce those neurotransmitters, the neurons need energy taken from your blood in the form of glucose. So, any exercise such as dance or aerobics classes that call for concentration, coordination, and skill also requires extra mental energy, which burns even more calories!

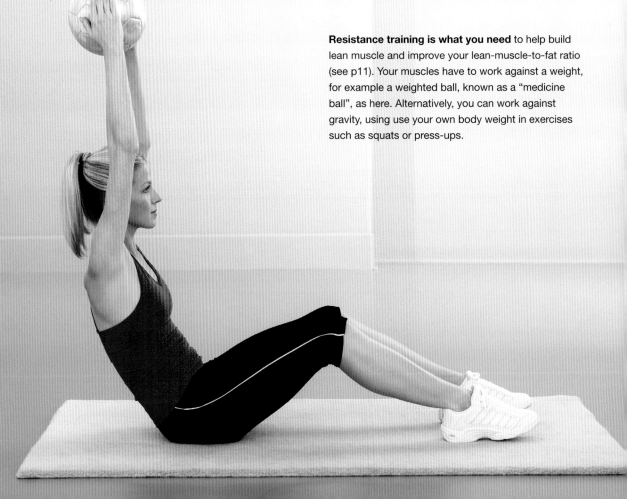

People often lose muscle as they age, partly because they're less active, so it's good to know that exercise, even when you're older, can reverse the muscle-loss process. When you're older, you can still get results, but you need to work harder for them than when your body was 10 years younger.

Help with staying active

So, if you don't want to gain weight, or if you want to lose it, the key is to increase your level of activity. You may need help to get you started or to keep you moving. If so, there are many professionals you can turn to.

A personal trainer is one. He or she may do some or a combination of the following, according to your needs: a thorough fitness assessment, a specially tailored exercise programme, make regular visits to work with you and check you're staying on track. Of course, a personal trainer is not a low-budget option.

A less expensive choice is to join a gym and work with an instructor there. He or she will show you how to use the various items of fitness equipment safely and will also assess your weight, your percentage of body fat (see p120), your lung capacity, and your flexibility. You'll be given a tailor-made fitness programme to follow, and every 6 to 8 weeks you can usually have a re-assessment, which will monitor your improvement. Then your fitness programme can be tweaked as required.

Seeing a good osteopath or physiotherapist can also be extremely helpful for getting you on the right track. He or she can identify any problem areas you might have – such as stiff knees or hips – or any that you might develop in the near future, for example if you spend all day hunched over a computer. Such advice is priceless as not only can

Resistance training is what you need to help build lean muscle and improve your lean-muscle-to-fat ratio (see p11). Your muscles have to work against a weight, for example a weighted ball, known as a "medicine ball", as here. Alternatively, you can work against gravity, using use your own body weight in exercises such as squats or press-ups.

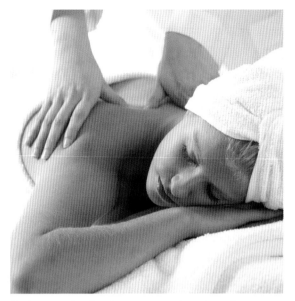

Seeing a professional masseur can be extremely beneficial. A massage helps to get rid of muscle tension, both before and after you work out, and is good for your circulation, too.

>> **boost the burn** exercise tips

- **Do resistance training.** Lean muscle mass burns calories (see p10) and resistance training helps build lean mass. The training works by overloading your muscles – making them perform so they're out of their comfort zone. Use weights or kettlebells at your gym – but be sure you have an induction so you know how to use them correctly. Alternatively, work with resistance bands at home.

- **Vary your exercise.** I've already said that if you don't vary your exercise, you'll reach a "plateau" (see p15). Then you'll find that you don't feel as satisfied at the end of your workout as you used to. You may also be gaining weight, even if you aren't eating more or exercising less. The reason is that your body has got used to that pattern of exercise, and has become more efficient as it anticipates your exercise programme. So try something else!

- **Add bursts of speed to any aerobic routine.** Known as interval training, this increases your heart rate, which then burns more calories. So, if you're walking, speed up for 20 or 30 seconds, then slow down for a minute or two. Repeat so you add two or three fast-paced intervals and gradually add longer, more intense intervals.

it stop you aggravating existing problems, but it can also help to prevent any condition you are unwittingly heading towards. Your osteopath or physiotherapist can also suggest the type of exercise that would suit you.

Exercise for every age

The World Health Organization defines fitness as "the ability to carry out daily tasks with alertness and efficiency whilst maintaining sufficient energy for leisure pursuits". If you're relatively fit, then this should describe you, and no matter how old you are, you can probably do most types of exercise. Yet some types of exercise may be slightly better for you at certain stages of your life.

Your 20s During our twenties most of us are so busy having fun that we don't realize what an easy ride we're having. We've only recently stopped growing, so our BMR is still relatively high, which means that a little exercise goes a long way.

At this age, you're usually fit enough for any form of exercise, so choose from high-impact cardio (like running and jogging), aerobic exercise, such as cycling or swimming, and resistance training, using your own body weight for doing exercises like squats, sit-ups, or press-ups, or using external resistance, such as a resistance band or free weights.

If you do have any specific issues you need to get to grips with, for example serious weight problems or particularly bad posture, now is the time to do it. Your body is still young and adaptable

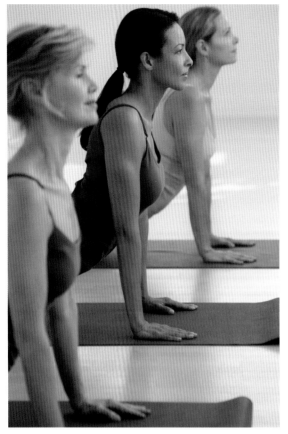

Yoga works whatever your age. The poses stimulate the hormone-secreting endocrine system and help to keep your muscles toned. Yoga's a great stress-buster, too.

and will respond more quickly to change. Make this a time to establish good exercise and eating habits.

Your 30s Between the ages of 28 and 32 is usually when most of us realize that our body "suddenly" isn't the same as it once was. Research has revealed that we naturally lose around 2kg (5lb) of lean body mass and replace it with fat every decade starting from our late 20s. Even if you weigh the same as you did in your 20s, chances are that fat has replaced some of your lean muscle.

Most gyms can take a body-fat reading, or you can buy a machine for home use. If you're female and aged between 20 and 39, a healthy body-fat reading is 21–33 per cent; between 40 and 59, the reading should be 23–34 per cent. If you *are* carrying extra fat, the longer it's there, the harder it

is to get rid of it. I'm a great believer in aerobic exercise as the best fat stripper, so whatever exercise you do, work aerobically in it, which means maintaining a steady pace for a long time.

If you haven't already started resistance training, now's a good time as your bones are already starting to become less dense and this, later in life, can lead to osteoporosis and fractures. Resistance training helps protect you against osteoporosis by slowing down the loss of minerals from your bones while building muscle, too.

Your 40s Whether or not you believe that the 40s are the new 30s, with all the resources we have at our disposal, there's no doubt that you can continue to feel and look great.

You may now need to start toning down your high-impact cardio (running and jogging) to low-impact (brisk walking, rowing, or using a cross trainer) to protect your knees. When walking, keep the aerobic pressure up by pumping your arms as you go or by holding hand weights. You may also want to work your core muscles, to keep – or encourage the return of – your nice flat tummy. Try targeted stomach exercises like crunches or planks, or go to a Pilates class. You should also continue – or start – resistance training exercise.

Also make sure you incorporate stretches in your exercise programme. These not only increase your range of movement, but will help tone your muscles. Yoga or Pilates are great for stretching.

Your 50s If you've reached your 50s and never exercised, remember, it's not too late, even though your metabolism will be slowing down (see p116). If you're a beginner, start by joining a gym and getting your fitness assessed so you're sure to work safely and within your capabilities.

Carry on – or start – resistance training to protect your bones, and do some low-impact cardio such as working on a rowing machine, swimming, or walking, especially uphill.

Finally, don't forget those stretches. If you're lucky, at this stage in your life, you may have more time for yourself, so you can focus on keeping your body in tip-top condition, both now and for many healthy decades to come.

Diet's important, too

As we've seen, calories are units of energy that we get from the food – the carbohydrates, fats, and protein – we eat (see p10). We take carbs in the form of sugars and complex carbs (bread, grains, beans, vegetables). Fat is usually sourced from oils, butter, meat, and cheese, but there are also high levels of fat in many junk foods, cakes, and biscuits. Protein is supplied by meat, poultry, fish, eggs, cheese, and by some beans and grains, but some of these protein sources also have high levels of fat, so you need to choose carefully.

As a general rule, most people need to take in *less* fat – particularly processed fats found in junk and processed foods – and *less* sugar, caffeine, and alcohol. And it would do most of us good to have *more* complex carbs, fibre (from fruit and vegetables), and water.

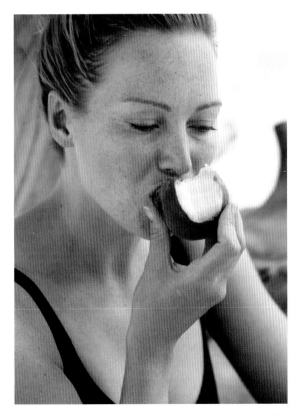

It's now recommended that one-third of your daily food should consist of fruit and vegetables. So there's truth in the old adage "an apple a day keeps the doctor away".

>> **boost the burn** eating tips

- **Eat protein.** Your BMR (see p10) rises after you eat because it takes energy to eat, digest, and metabolize your food. This is called "thermic effect". The thermic effect varies according to the type of food you eat. Proteins raise your BMR 30 per cent, carbohydrates raise it 6 per cent, while fats only raise it 4 per cent. Clearly, proteins win hands down!

- **Eat hot, spicy foods.** Foods containing chilli, horseradish, and mustard can also have a significant thermic effect, so eating those can raise your BMR.

- **Eat foods that contain iodine.** A diet that's low in iodine reduces your thyroid function, which slows your metabolism. The RDA (recommended daily allowance) is 150mcg. Foods that are richest in iodine are fish and shellfish, but if you happen to be allergic to these, consider taking a supplement. However, too much iodine is also bad for you, so only take a supplement on the advice of a professional practitioner.

- **Eat breakfast.** Your BMR is highest in the morning and tails off gradually through the day, so take advantage of this daily peak. An American study showed that eating a proper meal at the start of the day boosted BMR by 10 per cent and that people who skipped breakfast or lunch had a lower BMR than those who didn't.

- **Don't go on a crash diet.** If you eat too little, your metabolism slows so your body can conserve the energy it's got. Crash dieting can reduce your BMR as much as 15 per cent. Crash dieting also means you lose lean muscle tissue, which in turn reduces your BMR.

>> **broaden** your horizons

Working out in your living room is convenient and is a good place to start, but if your body craves new ways to exercise, you'll probably want to broaden your horizons. The world out there is full of great opportunities for taking your exercise on to the next stage.

Carry on with the good work at home, but now try and make exercise part of your life on a regular basis. Here are some ideas for doing that.

Get out

If you've had fun doing the Running Workout, you may want to run or jog outdoors. The mistake most people make when they start running is going too fast, and that simply makes them give up. My favourite tip for beginners is "walk a lampost, run a lampost". In other words, run from one lampost to the next, then walk between the following two. When that feels comfortable, and you're ready to push yourself a bit further, try running two lamposts and walking one. If you start to get out of breath, you can always walk two and run one, but be sure to pick up your pace again as soon as you can.

If you're unfit, are carrying a lot of extra weight or have any lower back, knee, or hip problems, it's best to start "low-impact" – marching or walking instead of running or jogging. And if you are older, try walking fast with handweights or walking uphill rather than running. Both will give you a workout that's as intense as jogging or running.

Get in a pool

Swimming's a great form of exercise as it burns calories without putting any stress on your joints. The water takes the strain, supporting 90 per cent of your body weight. Doing the crawl is an especially good calorie burner.

But if swimming's not for you, then try aqua aerobics. Essentially, this is aerobic exercise (see p11) in water. Again, the water supports a large part of your body weight, even though you're exercising in shallow water. A typical class will have you marching, walking and running forwards and back, jumping – even doing cross-country ski moves. It's just like doing my Running Workout (see pp70–81), but in water.

Go to a gym

Going to a gym gives you the chance to work with different types of equipment. It also helps you to vary the type of exercise you do, which is good for

---

> ## >> **tips for** your next stage
>
> - **When you're outdoors,** run on grass rather than concrete. The strain on your knees will be far less. You'll definitely notice the difference.
>
> - **When you go to the gym,** have an induction by one of the instructors. That way you'll use the equipment safely. You can also ask the instructor to devise a programme that's tailor-made for you.
>
> - **When you join a class,** try to watch one first to be sure it's right for you. Most clubs and lesiure centres allow this.

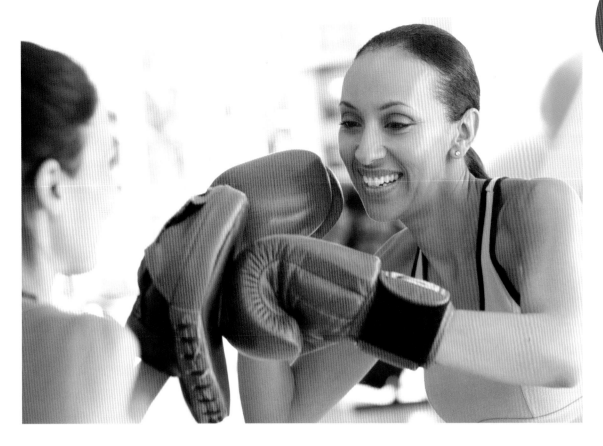

burning calories. If it's more running that you want, you can run on a treadmill, perhaps adjusting the gradient so you can walk "uphill". Other gym equipment that will give you a good cardio workout – one that raises your heart rate, which is good for burning calories – includes stationary bikes, rowing machines, elliptical walkers (also called cross trainers), and stair masters.

Gyms offer a range of strength and resistance training equipment, too. These build muscle and strengthen bones, so helping to guard against osteoporosis. Different machines are designed to work different parts of the body, and you can also work with free weights and kettlebells.

Join a class

If you're ready to take your dancing, aerobics, or boxing to the next level, joining a class is the way to go. Dance classes come in many shapes and forms, from ballroom, to salsa, to hip-hop. They're

Boxing is becoming more and more popular with women. Boxing with a sparring partner or a punchbag will burn an average 165 calories per 15 minutes.

great fun and a good way of meeting people. Alternatively, go along with a group of friends and burn calories together.

There are also many styles of aerobics classes, but all involve doing routines to music, just like my *15 Minute Calorie Burn* workouts. As you'll have discovered, this is great for helping your motivation and coordination.

And last but by no means least, there are gyms devoted solely to boxing and boxing training. After your 15 minute "taster" you may feel you want to get some boxing gloves on and start punching something. Or you might like to try kickboxing classes – similar to boxing, but using martial arts-style kicks, which give you a good lower-body workout, as well as burning loads of calories.

useful resources

Most of these resources are my personal recommendations and will give you a starting point in areas that you may wish to explore further. It is often difficult to find really good health professionals. Those listed here are people I work with regularly who are great at what they do.

general fitness resources

bbc.co.uk/health
bbc.co.uk/health/healthy_living/fitness/
Useful general website with features on the benefits of being fit, how to choose the appropriate type of exercise and finding out how much exercise you need to stay healthy.

The Register of Exercise Professionals (REPs)
8–10 Crown Hill
Croydon
Surrey CR0 1RZ
exerciseregister.org
Tel: +44 (0) 20 8686 6464
National register of exercise professionals in the U.K. Set up to help safeguard and promote the health and interests of people who are using the services of exercise and fitness instructors, teachers, and trainers. This is a good place to start if you're looking for a fitness instructor.

osteopathy, massage, and acupuncture

Clive D. Lathey
Osteopath
The Putney Clinic
1 Deodar Road
London SW15 2NP
putneyclinic.co.uk
Tel: +44 (0) 20 8789 3881

K J W Osteopathy
221 Westbourne Park Road
London W11 1EA
kjw-osteopathy.co.uk
Tel: +44 (0) 20 7243 0007

Cinzia Scorzon
Acupuncturist and homeopath
18 St. Albans Place
London N1 0NX
Tel: +44 (0) 20 7288 2999
cinziascorzon@gmail.com

Petra Thamm
Tel: +44 (0) 7879 401 342
Specialist for sports massage and soft-tissue injuries.

gyms

KX Gym
151 Draycott Ave
London SW3 3AL
kxgym.co.uk
Tel: +44 (0) 20 7584 5333
Home of London's top experts in nutrition, strength, and conditioning.

Stephen Price Gym
3 Jubilee Place
London SW3 3TD
stephen-price.com
Tel: +44 (0) 20 7351 3332

YMCA England
640 Forest Road
London E17 3D
www.ymca.org.uk
The largest single voluntary sector organization offering a wide range of individual and group services including exercise classes and fitness studios that are accessible and inclusive for people of all ages and skill levels. The website has a search facility to help you find your nearest YMCA.

running

Runners Need
runnersneed.co.uk
Tel: +44 (0) 20 7278 948
Specialist London stockists of
running shoes and all running
accessories; expert advice. Also
has an online shop.

dancing

Bar Salsa
96 Charing Cross Road
London WC2H OJG
Tel: +44 (0) 20 7379 3277
barsalsa.eu
Salsa club and bar. Offers
lessons for beginners.

Dance Works
16 Balderton Street
London W1K 6TN
danceworks.co.uk
Tel: +44 (0) 20 7629 6183
Opened in 1982, with six studios
and offering a large selection of
dance, fitness, and martial arts
classes.

Pineapple Studios
7 Langley Street
Covent Garden
London WC2H 9JA
pineapple.uk.com
Tel: +44 (0) 20 7836 4004
Dance studios with sprung floors,
mirrors, barres, music systems,
and pianos. Classes for
beginners to professionals in
ballet, ballroom, street, jazz,
salsa, tap, and more.

boxing and kickboxing

Beyond Fighting
beyondfighting.com
Leeds' largest martial arts club,
offering classes, private tuition,
and personalized e-learning
programmes in kickboxing and
martial arts.

Bob Breen Academy
16 Hoxton Square
London N1 6NT
Tel: +44 (0) 20 7729 5789
bobbreen.com
Gym offering boxing, Thai
boxing, and kickboxing

Combat Shotokan
combatshotokan.co.uk
Club in Aberdeen, offering martial
arts and personal safety tuition.

Karmaa
101 The Stables Market
Chalk Farm Road
London NW1 8AH
karmaa.co.uk/index.htm
Tel: +44 (0) 20 7485 7474
Gym offering kickboxing,
martial arts.

K O Gyms
ko-muaythai.com
A chain of London gyms offering
Thai boxing and kickboxing.

Paragon Gym
6–8 Boundary Street
Shoreditch
London E2 7JE
paragongym.co.uk
Tel: +44 (0) 207 256 0990
Runs classes in boxing and
kickboxing.

equipment

Fitness Mad
Units 2–4 Willersey Industrial
Estate
Willersey
Worcs WR12 7RR
fitness-mad.com
Tel: +44 (0) 1386 859 551
Specializes in products for
resistance and strength-training.

Newitt & Co. Ltd.
Claxton Hall
Flaxton
York
North Yorks YO60 7RE
newitts.com
Family firm offering sports
equipment by mail order. Supplier
of gym balls and exercise mats.

Niketown London
236 Oxford Street
London W1N 9DF
Tel: +44 (0) 20 7612 0800
For all sports clothing and
accessories.

Physical Company
physicalcompany.co.uk
Offers fitness and gym
equipment online and by
mail order.

Powerhouse Fitness
powerhouse-fitness.co.uk
Offers a wide range of gym and
sports equipment.

index

acknowledgments

Author's acknowledgments
Thanks to all my family for their support, and for putting up with me through all my never-ending projects ... Mum, Dad, Jazzie, Jessye, Mahlon, and Maia. You make all things possible. Corny but true.

Big up Dagmar, Ricky, Bunty, Kate, Tracy, Dianne, Rodney, Aitch, Chrystelle, Janet, and Anita. Thanks for listening or at least doing a good job of pretending to!

Thanks to Joey Dubens for being there since the start and encouraging me to the end.

Thanks to Brigsy for the most important thing on any job – makeup!

Big swoosh of a thank you to Kemi at Nike, South Africa and to Stephanie and Jumoke at Nike, London.

Thank you to all the DK crew.

To Borra Garson, a big thank you with low-fat cream and cherries on top!

Publisher's acknowledgments
Dorling Kindersley thanks photographer Ruth Jenkinson and her assistant Carly Churchill; sweatyBetty for the loan of exercise clothing; Viv Riley at Touch Studios; the model Carla Collins; Rachel Jones and Brigitta Smart for the hair and makeup; Peter Kirkham for proofreading; Hilary Bird for the index.

Picture Credits
The publisher would like to thank the following for their kind permission to reproduce their photographs:
Corbis: Comstock 119; Cathrine Wessel 11; Getty Images: Image Source 12; Tetra Images 120; Photolibrary: Stockbroker 123

All other images © Dorling Kindersley
For further information see: www.dkimages.com

about Efua Baker

Efua (pronounced "Ef'wah") started her professional life as a dancer and fashion model. For the past 15 years she has been a ground-breaking personal trainer or "body sculptor", as she prefers to be called. The focus of her London-based practice has always been to ensure her clients look good and feel great.

Efua has gained a loyal following in the image-driven world of celebrity where her unique and highly effective "body turnaround " techniques are much sought-after.

Efua doesn't just work with famous bodies, she has also developed exercise and motivational programmes for large and diverse groups including new mums, youngsters, and even entire families. It's fair to say she has worked with every type of body there is!

Her workout style draws from many disciplines including dance, body-building, martial arts, yoga, and boxing. Her motto is, "No matter who you are, you are only ever one workout away from looking better and feeling amazing."